ALL MEDICINES ARE POISON!

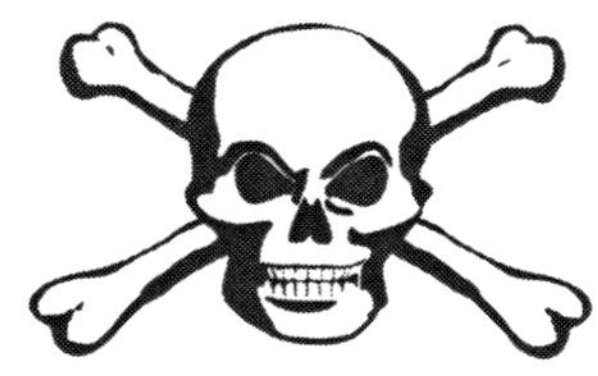

Making Your Way through the Medical Minefield

With your guide

MELVIN H. KIRSCHNER, MPH, MD

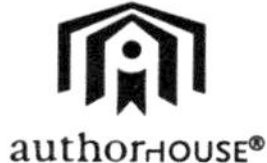

authorHOUSE®

AuthorHouse™
1663 Liberty Drive
Bloomington, IN 47403
www.authorhouse.com
Phone: 1-800-839-8640

First published by AuthorHouse 8/31/2009

ISBN: 978-1-4490-1165-9 (sc)
ISBN: 978-1-4490-1164-2 (hc)

Library of Congress Control Number: 2009908297

Printed in the United States of America
Bloomington, Indiana

This book is printed on acid-free paper.

Cover design and interior illustrations by Darin Kirschner.

ACKNOWLEDGEMENTS

I would probably never have written this book, if it had not been for my professors at the University of Southern California School of Medicine many years ago. Two in particular had a profound influence on me as a medical student and also the way I practiced medicine and cared for patients during the 47 years I was in family practice.

The title of the book reflects a comment made to us by Dr. John Webb during his pharmacology course. Dr. Telfer Reynolds, our internal medicine professor, was a constant taskmaster and an endless fountain of medical knowledge. After I went into practice, I often attended medical meetings that Professor Reynolds conducted. He always remembered my name and years later came, at my request, for a consultation on a patient whom I had hospitalized because of perplexing symptoms.

My dedication list would be incomplete if I didn't thank Marty Rich, a dear friend, who read through and corrected several revisions of this book in order to correct syntax and content so that the average lay person would not be harassed by medical jargon.

Melvin H Kirschner, MPH, MD

PREFACE

Everything we do has a risk-benefit ratio. When I graduated from the UCLA School of Public Health, I went to work for the Tulare County Health Department as a health inspector (sanitarian). In those days, the county required we drive our own car at work, so I bought my very first car, a new 1949 Plymouth. One day, the local newspaper reported the Tulare Parachute Loft was selling their surplus of new airplane seat belts. In those days, cars did not come equipped with seat belts. I bought two seat belts and installed them in my new car. Thereafter, whenever I had a passenger, I'd say, "Buckle up for safety." Several years later, all cars came with seat belts.

Driving or riding in a car has a risk-benefit ratio. But it's necessary for us to drive or ride, so we take that risk. The seat belts lower the risk, but don't eliminate it. When we become sick, we sometimes take medicines to reduce the discomfort and duration of the illness, but all medicines have potential side effects and risks. The patient and doctor must weigh the benefit of a treatment before taking the risk of any side effects that might occur.

This book explores many facets of this and related health care issues drawn from a lifetime of experience in public health and family practice. The book is derived from lectures, debates, articles, Op-Ed pieces, letters to the editor, and essays I have written during almost sixty years of service in the American health care system. I have rewritten them as individual essays. I have tried to arrange them in a rational sequence of subjects and removed as many redundancies as I could without losing the flow of the individual essay. But some redundancies remain. I hope the reader will not find this annoying, but will realize I want each essay to be able to stand alone.

TABLE OF CONTENTS

BE AN INFORMED HEALTH CARE CONSUMER

ALL MEDICINES ARE POISON

When I was in the second year of medical school in the 1950s, we were taught about medicines and pharmacology. At the University of Southern California (USC), we were very fortunate to have a pharmacology professor of world stature, Dr. John L. Webb. During our first year, while we were learning our basic medical sciences, he was visiting Maoist Red China, studying traditional Chinese medicines. Able to speak fluent Chinese, he was one of the rare Americans invited to China during the Mao era. We met him for the first time as we assembled for our initial class in pharmacology.

The setting was somewhat strange. At that time, the new medical school campus was just starting construction across the street from Los Angeles County General Hospital. Most of our classes were held in the old chemistry building at the main USC campus, which was across town from the planned new medical school location. The old chemistry building was so overcrowded that the pharmacology class had to be held in the cavernous general assembly auditorium on campus. It was designed to accommodate at least a thousand students.

In those days, our medical school class of fifty-eight was mostly male. There were only three female students. Today, medical school classes at USC are split about fifty-fifty. We were seated in a dimly lit corner of the large auditorium. Professor Webb was on the stage, standing behind a brightly lit lectern. He presented a rather commanding figure as he looked down at us for the first time.

"Ladies and gentlemen," he said, "I am here to teach you how to poison people!"

A brief pause followed while we sat stunned by those words. We were expecting to learn how to cure people, not poison them.

Then he added, "Without killing them, of course."

Thus, the title of this book originates from Dr. Webb's introduction to pharmacology. There followed a discussion of why and how all medicines are poison in some situations. I have never forgotten that lesson in the more than fifty years since I heard that statement. Years of medical practice have validated repeatedly what Dr. Webb taught us about medicines. Throughout that semester, he taught us to appreciate the uses and benefits that medicines have, but also the burdens (adverse reactions) they could cause and their interactions with other substances.

Properly used medicines are of great benefit and save lives, but we must always be aware of the burdens. Furthermore anything we ingest can cause problems. With this benefits-versus-burdens relationship in mind, we make our health decisions. Physicians are expected to educate patients about these matters. In our society, doctors advise, and patients decide.

When I was a child, tincture of iodine came in a unique brown bottle with a skull and crossbones embossed on its side. The skull and crossbones implied danger, poison, and even death. In those days, tincture of iodine was widely used as an antiseptic for cuts and abrasions. It stung when it was applied, but not from the iodine. The sting was from the alcohol it contained. It was painted on cuts and lacerations to keep them from becoming infected. Iodine is still used, but in an aqueous solution that is still an excellent antiseptic. Without alcohol as the solvent, it doesn't burn when applied to a wound.

In the tincture of iodine days, we kids preferred Mercurochrome. It could be applied to a wound without causing the burning pain that iodine caused. It also prevented infection, and it wasn't marked as poison. In fact, Mercurochrome was a mercury compound, and it was a poison, but the bottle did not have a skull and crossbones embossed on it. The likelihood of actually becoming poisoned by the mercury in Mercurochrome was remote. One used a small amount on the wound, and it was never ingested.

Humans have used mercury in many forms. Thiomersal, an organic mercury compound, was used for many years as a preservative of drugs in sterile ampules (small glass bottles) that held several doses prior to injection. Some authorities suspected thiomersal in immunizing vaccines was causing autism in children.[1] The Food and Drug Administration (FDA) has ordered that thiomersal be removed from injectable medications. Studies have shown that thiomersal does not cause autism, but this chemical substance has never found its way back into pediatric immunization vaccines. They now do not contain mercury.

Another mercury hazard exists in certain fish that feed in mercury-contaminated waters. The FDA and Environmental Protection Agency (EPA) have jointly issued a warning suggesting to the public (and especially pregnant women) to avoid eating certain fish that contain excessive amounts of mercury.[2] The list includes shark, swordfish, tilefish, and king mackerel. These fish are known to concentrate the ingested mercury in their flesh. In theory, eating large quantities of these varieties

---

1 CDC, "Mercury and Vaccines."

2 EPA-823-R-04005, "What You Need to Know about Mercury in Fish and Shellfish," March 2004.

of fish may present a hazard. It doesn't seem to bother the fish. By my calculation, one would need to eat an awfully lot of mercury-contaminated fish over a long period to reach a dangerous level of poisoning. Recently, pregnant women and children have been especially advised to limit their consumption of tuna. This information is detailed on the Internet at the FDA's Web site.

Another issue widely discussed in the dental literature, is the use of amalgams to fill cavities in teeth. Amalgams are compounded with mercury. Some dentists advocate removing all the amalgams and replacing them with mercury-free substances. This practice is based on the theory that the mercury in the amalgam is slowly absorbed from the tooth into the patient's body, thus causing a toxic reaction. Most dentists do not believe this because mercury poisoning has not been demonstrated in people who have had amalgams in their fillings for many years. The American Dental Association (ADA) and most dentists regard it as unnecessary to replace amalgams with fillings that do not contain mercury.

The National Council Against Health Fraud (NCAHF) published a position paper on the subject of amalgams on its Web site at www.ncahf.org. The dentists on the board of the NCAHF agree with the Council's position paper, which recommends against the removal of fillings containing mercury.

Iodine and mercury are two examples of natural substances that have been found beneficial in one setting but present risks and burdens that must be considered when they are used for other purposes.

WHAT YOU NEED TO KNOW ABOUT THE FDA

Prior to 1906, when the Pure Food and Drug Act came into existence, the use of medications by patients and doctors was essentially a buyer-beware market. Hucksters could sell anything and make any statement about the use and contents of their products, whether true or false.

Journalists of the time and books such as *The Jungle* by Upton Sinclair influenced Congress. The book vividly described the terrible sanitation and contamination of the food products the meatpacking industry of the time was producing. A complete copy of this text is still available on the Internet more than one hundred years since it was first published. In response to the poor sanitation and purity of the food being produced at the time, Congress created the FDA in 1906. This agency's mandate was to see that foods and drugs were not adulterated or misbranded.

In 1912, Congress added an amendment that specifically prohibited "false and fraudulent" curative or therapeutic claims on the label. In 1938, the Federal

Food, Drug, and Cosmetic Act was passed. For the first time, the FDA required that, before marketing a new drug, a manufacturer had to submit evidence that the drug was safe and effective.

ANOTHER STEP TOWARD PATIENT SAFETY

The Kefauver-Harris Amendment of 1962 represented another major step forward for patient safety. Among other requirements, the Kefauver-Harris Amendment mandated the inclusion of complete professional information in virtually all prescription drug packages and sales literature distributed to physicians.

At that time, I had been in practice for only two years. As a new doctor, I found the description of hazards, side effects, and precautions to be very helpful in prescribing safely and appropriately. Detailed descriptions now accompany all prescription medicines. They are known as "package inserts," and they are extremely complex and somewhat confusing. Doctors have been accused of not reading them carefully enough before prescribing a new medication, so the FDA is currently in the process of revising the format so important prescribing information, such as adverse reactions and interactions, are displayed more prominently and made easier for physicians to review.

I read and reread this information and carry a pocket prescription drug reference (pocket PDR) with me at all times, yet the prescriptions I write still sometimes cause unanticipated adverse reactions. The number of humans studied during the required pre-release research period is relatively small. When millions of people start to use a new medicine after it is released for general use, unexpected side effects, interactions, and hazards surface.

For this reason, in the 1970s, the Drug Quality Reporting System (DQRS) was established, and pharmacists and physicians began reporting adverse reactions. The information garnered from these reports makes it possible for the FDA to monitor and even recall products that prove to be unsafe after their release.

THE STANDARD DRUG APPROVAL PROCESS

Drug companies spend millions of dollars researching new products. The company that is first to market a new class of medication is likely to make more profits than later competitors are. The drug approval process was tediously slow. This was necessitated by the methods required by the FDA to assure new drugs reach the market only after careful and thorough evaluation.

The FDA's Center for Drug Evaluation and Research (CDER) requires a standard protocol for studying potentially new drugs. Each proposed new substance is first subjected to animal studies in at least two species. This pharmacology/toxicology testing is to develop adequate data to undergird a decision that it is reasonably safe to proceed with human trials.

The first human clinical studies (Phase I) may be conducted in patients, and they are usually done in human volunteers. These studies, usually conducted on twenty to eighty subjects, are designed to evaluate drug metabolism and mechanism of action in humans. Side effects of increasing doses are also evaluated at this phase.

Phase II includes controlled clinical studies that are conducted to obtain preliminary data on the effectiveness of the drug for a particular indication in patients with the disease or condition. This phase of testing also helps determine the common short-term effects and risks associated with the drug. Phase II studies usually involve several hundred people.

If the Phase II studies do not eliminate a new drug, it then goes on to Phase III. These clinical studies are intended to gather additional information about effectiveness and safety that is needed to evaluate the overall benefit-risk relationship of the drug. Phase III studies also provide information for inclusion in the product brochure being prepared for doctors who will be prescribing the new drug. This phase usually includes several hundred to several thousand people.

The real test of a drug is when it is approved for marketing and millions of patients use it. The FDA is aware that no amount of careful preapproval testing will reveal all of the risks and adverse reactions. So physicians are encouraged to report adverse reactions and effects not already described in the product brochure that accompanies prescription drugs.

When such reports are made, the FDA evaluates their frequency and significance. Reports of a serious nature have resulted in the addition of a black box warning to the product brochures and, at times, recall of the drug from the market. Side effects appear in the adverse reactions section of the brochure.

Enlisting adequate numbers of qualified volunteers for clinical trials has been a problem. In the past, clinical trials have primarily been done at the university clinics, but, in recent years, community-based physicians have done much research. Unfortunately, unscrupulous individuals have sometimes failed to follow the rigid requirements of valid research. Some well-meaning physicians who have been asked to participate in clinical trials or refer their patients do not understand the ethics involved.

The Los Angeles County Medical Association/Bar Association Joint Committee on Biomedical Ethics developed "Guidelines for Physicians Participating in Clinical Trials."[3] With these guidelines, the committee hopes to provide a set of ethical standards that can be followed so physicians understand their ethical role and the patient is neither harmed nor misinformed.

These guidelines made it very clear that issues of informed consent, privacy, institutional review committee oversight, and other safeguards are in place before any human experimentation can be done in this society. This is a very touchy subject, which involves medical ethics, as all of the Committee's guidelines do.

An e-mail newsletter addressed primarily to physicians, "ePocrates Clinical Trials Connection," discussed the issue of clinical trials, stating that 80 percent of all trials are delayed due to poor recruitment. According to ePocrates News, in 2001, there were twelve hundred drugs in Phase III clinical trials. Only twenty-four new drugs and twenty-seven new drug formulations or combinations were approved that year.[4]

CDER monitors study design and conduct of clinical trials to ensure people in the trials are not exposed to unnecessary risks.

---

3 Los Angeles County Medical Association/Bar Association Joint Committee on Biomedical Ethics, "Guidelines for Doctors Who Do Clinical Trials."

4 ePocrates, "Clinical Trials Connection," September 2002.

I will later discuss informed consent, a critical component of all treatment and medical care in the United States. Obtaining the patient's informed consent is also required for clinical trial research. This requirement originates from the patient's legal and ethical right to direct what happens to his or her body. The language used to obtain consent must be in clearly understandable lay terminology.

THE PRACTICE OF FAST TRACKING

Another factor has entered the equation in recent years. The public has been demanding that drugs that show promise of helping critically and seriously ill patients be released before the required comprehensive studies are completed. This is commonly known as "fast tracking."

I agree with this practice, as the patients on whose behalf this is done are dying or suffering terribly and grasping at straws. But I do object to fast tracking drugs that are rushed to market before the benefits and side effects are well studied and understood solely because early release promotes profits.

Please don't read me wrong. Patients have greatly benefited from the many wonderful new medications that this industry has produced. But, as a physician, I must think of patient welfare first. I do not believe it is necessary to hasten a new drug to market when the condition it is intended to treat isn't life threatening or other effective medicines already exist.

Obviously, diseases such as AIDS, metastatic cancer, and other illnesses that lead to a painful and miserable death prompted the development of fast track standards. The language in the fast track rules that permitted other medications intended to treat nonfatal conditions to attain fact track status is in this statement that I quote from the FDA's fact track requirements:

> The fast track programs of the FDA are designed to facilitate the development and expedite review of new drugs that are intended to treat serious or life-threatening conditions and that demonstrate the potential to address unmet medical needs.

The phrase "unmet medical needs" opens a broad spectrum of possible conditions for which new drugs could (and should) be developed, but not, in my opinion, via the fast track route. The fast track approval route does bring drugs to market sooner than the normal FDA approval route does. This could bring life-saving drugs to market, which might be used in AIDS and terminal cancer, where their absence would result in certain death anyway. If such a drug failed to work or even hastened death, the patient might still have an option to use it, hoping some benefit might be derived where none had existed. But, in a nonfatal illness, where no useful medications exist, the best interests of patients require the usual, more time-consuming, complete FDA protocol.

Since the fast track protocol has existed, several medicines for nonfatal conditions have reached the market prematurely. Subsequent experience, such as unexpected patient deaths attributed to the new medicine, has required their withdrawal from the market. This has occasionally happened with drugs that reach the market after the standard, more time-consuming approval route, but I believe fast tracking increases the risk of the occurrence of unexpected adverse reactions. Congress tried to make fast track safer by increasing the numbers of FDA staff personnel who are responsible for overseeing the drug's approval. The pharmaceutical industry was required to pay extra fees when a fast track request was sanctioned. Presumably, the increased revenue that permitted the FDA to add more staff to the evaluation team of the drug on the fast track will speed up the process without sacrificing the quality of the evaluation.

HOW DRUGS ARE CLASSIFIED

Over the years, I have seen drugs come to market and then be withdrawn. I have seen medications changed from easily obtained, non-prescription to prescription. I have seen legal substances made illegal. To understand how and why all this occurs, we need to understand how the FDA and Drug Enforcement Agency (DEA) categorize medicines in this country.

The various food and drug rules come from two places: Congress and regulations promulgated by the government agencies that enforce congressional laws.

The DEA oversees the following set of categories.[5] All substances used as medicines fall into one of these five categories. They are designated as "schedules" by the DEA, but doctors generally use the descriptive word "class."

SCHEDULE I (CLASS I): ILLEGAL SUBSTANCES

Substances that are currently illegal to use include lysergic acid, peyote, heroin, and marijuana. In the last few years, several states— California, Washington,

5 A wealth of information about DEA functions is cited on the Internet.

Oregon, Alaska, Maine, Hawaii, Colorado, Nevada, Vermont, and Montana—had already voted the sale and use of medical marijuana legal. Other states have indicated they will follow this trend, but the federal government was contesting such use.

To placate the federal demands that sellers and users of medical marijuana be punished, states where it had been voted legal were only gently slapping the hands that used it for legitimate medical reasons by levying a small fine.

As I write this, President Obama's newly appointed attorney general announced the United States would not prosecute medical pot sales.[6]

SCHEDULE II (CLASS II): DRUGS LIKELY TO CAUSE ADDICTION

This schedule/class consists of substances and drugs that are prone to cause addiction, including cocaine, morphine, amphetamines, barbiturates, and various other substances deemed to be addictive or prone to abuse, are also in Class II. Doctors may legally prescribe or use these medicines, but, in some states, the physician must apply for a controlled drug license number. Written prescriptions must be on special duplicate or triplicate,

6 "U.S. Won't Prosecute Medical Pot Sales," *Los Angeles Times*, 19 March 2009.

sequentially numbered prescription form pads that are difficult to forge or copy. They must also be imprinted with the doctor's name, narcotic license number, and office location. In California, where I practiced, a more comprehensive program replaced the triplicate requirement on January 1, 2005. The new controlled drug plan covered a much more extensive list of medications than before. All of which were considered to be drugs of abuse, regardless of class. These medications must be written on the specially printed form that cannot be copied. But the people who abuse drugs always seem to find a way to beat the system.

Within two months from the beginning of this program, a wary pharmacist faxed a prescription to me that he doubted I had written. It was on official paper with my DEA number, but neither the address printed on it nor the handwriting was mine. Somebody had forged prescriptions resembling mine on this official form that could not be copied. The forger must have gotten to someone at the print shop that produced my forms. There's no telling how many of these bogus prescription blanks were successfully used before this observant pharmacist discovered the forgery. The pharmacist made a report to the police and DEA and alerted me.

After passing these bogus prescriptions at several different drug stores, another pharmacist recognized the prescription was a fake. He immediately called the police and me. The individual, who was waiting for the phony prescription to be filled, was finally arrested for attempting to pass a forged prescription. Since then, another incident of forgeries of my controlled drug prescriptions has become known, but the culprit has yet to be apprehended. If this has happened to my practice twice, who knows how many other doctors have had the same experience?

Although the misuse of narcotics have troubled me, I believe most addicts are ill and need to be treated rather than be punished. Our prisons are full of people arrested for illegal narcotic possession. Many people apparently sell narcotics in order to support their habit. In my view, the real criminals are the pushers who propagate this ugly practice solely for profit.

SCHEDULE III (CLASS III): DRUGS THAT MAY BE ABUSED

This schedule/class contains drugs that may possibly be abused, but they are considered to be less likely to cause addiction than the medicines in Class II. This group of medicines includes many milder sleeping pills, pain pills, and tranquilizers that California physicians could prescribe on an ordinary prescription blank until the 2005 law was passed. All of these medications are now controlled in California and require the special prescription forms that were discussed previously.

SCHEDULE IV (CLASS IV): UNLIKELY TO BE ABUSED, BUT REQUIRE SUPERVISION

This schedule/class includes blood pressure-lowering drugs, antibiotics, and other substances that might be hazardous if used in an unsupervised way. They require a doctor's examination and prescription. They may also require laboratory tests or other tests, such as x-rays and/or electrocardiography. They are likely to require specific doses and different frequency of use, depending on the patient's body mass, age, and intensity of the illness. The DEA requires a physician's prescription because patients should not be taking these medicines without a doctor's supervision.

SCHEDULE V (CLASS V): LOW POTENTIAL FOR ABUSE

These products are subject to state and local requirements. Some may be obtained without a doctor's prescription in a low-dosage formulation. Then they are known as over-the-counter (OTC) medicines. The stronger dosage formulations may require a doctor's prescription. One example is ibuprofen. It's OTC formulation is at two hundred milligrams, but it requires a prescription for the four hundred, six hundred, or eight hundred milligram tablet.

While many OTC substances are relatively safe to use, many, such as aspirin, vitamin D, and iron compounds, can cause toxic effects when used in excessive doses. Excessive use of non-prescription analgesics and anti-inflammatory drugs can cause ulcers, kidney damage, or even liver toxicity.

SUBSTANCES LIMITED TO USE BY SPECIFIC MEDICAL SPECIALISTS

In the 1960s, thalidomide was already on the market in Europe, but it was still in clinical trials in the United States. The FDA banned the drug because it was causing birth defects, especially limb dysplasia known as phocomelia. This word is derived from phocomelus, a creature with very short arms and legs. People with phocomelia have one or more short limbs. Their hands and feet seem to be pathologically attached directly to their bodies.

Since the early 1960s, when the FDA kept thalidomide from being marketed in the United States, I have seen a number of other drugs reinstated after they had been taken off the market for dangerous effects. Forty years after being removed from consideration, thalidomide was approved for limited use by specially licensed physicians. The drug still bears a warning prohibiting its use in pregnant women.

Other drugs on the market increase the risk of birth defects, but their use is very restricted. Physicians are expected to prescribe them to premenopausal women only after carefully considering the necessity, risks, and benefits. The best example is Accutane, which requires laboratory tests to assure the patient is not pregnant and a written agreement to avoid pregnancy while taking the medicine. A release signed by the patient is required before it can be prescribed. The Accutane black box also illustrates a figure of a pregnant female with a strike out X over it. This is an example of how detailed and explicit a black box warning can become.

All of the barriers and complications related to obtaining a prescription for Accutane might cause the reader to suspect it's addicting or severely habit-forming or perhaps cures a rare and serious disease. It's not! It's for the treatment of acne. However, in all fairness to people who suffer from this minor cosmetic condition, they often live a tortured life of self-depreciation and are willing to take almost any risk to control their acne.

THE INCREASING FREQUENCY OF MEDICINE RECALLS

In the last ten years, several medications, some of which I had prescribed in the past, were removed from the marketplace.[7] One of these medicines had been prescribed for me as a patient, and I suffered side effects from its use. Adverse reaction reports that practicing physicians sent to the FDA after the release of a medicine could result in a decision to withdraw it from the marketplace. The pre-market studies involve a few thousand subjects. As the reader is aware, once a drug reaches the market, millions of subjects will use the medicine. It's then that unacceptable adverse reactions and even deaths are more likely to come to the FDA's attention.

One of the drugs withdrawn from the market was Oraflex, an anti-inflammatory, because it had caused serious liver and kidney damage in some patients. It was released in the early 1980s, about the same time as Motrin. Although Oraflex is long gone, Motrin is still on the market. It is now an OTC drug, as the generic medication ibuprofen. The few patients for whom I had prescribed Oraflex before it was withdrawn lauded it as

---

7 Seventeen drugs have been withdrawn from the market in nine years: Tysabri, Vioxx, Duragesic, Ephedra, Baycol, Raplon, Duract, Posicor, Rezulin, Fen-Phen, Pondimin, Redux, Seldane, Hismanal, Propulsid, and Lotronix (http://www.yourlawyer.com/newsletter/read/9).

a wonderful solution for their arthritic aches and pains. They had reported no side effects. They were terribly disappointed when I could no longer write prescriptions for their medicine.

We now know that this entire family of nonsteroidal anti-inflammatory drugs (NSAIDs) are capable of doing this and more. I have seen two of my patients bleed severely from ulcers caused by the NSAIDs I had prescribed for them. I saw an elderly woman bleed to death in an emergency room from an ulcer caused by an NSAID. This happened despite every effort by the emergency room team to save her life. That particular NSAID is still available on the prescription market because it is perceived that its benefits outweigh the risks.

Unfortunately, it sometimes takes journal articles and news reports to precipitate the withdrawal action. Both Vioxx and Bextra, potent and effective anti-inflammatory medicines, suffered that fate. The other alternative has been to restrict prescription of these drugs by rheumatologists only.

The FDA has withdrawn drugs and then returned them to the market for use by a specified group of physicians. Lotronix is useful for irritable bowel syndrome. The FDA took it off the market because it caused problems and even death in some elderly women. It was eventually returned to the market, but only gastroenterologists can prescribe it now. More recently, Zelnorm, a drug with similar use as Lotronix, was taken off the market because it may have caused heart problems and strokes in some patients. It was also returned to the market for limited use by gastroenterologists.

When I graduated from medical school, many fewer specialists were in this country. General practitioners wrote most of the prescriptions. But there also were many fewer drugs to study and prescribe competently. Specialists are trained in a very narrow segment of medical practice. They become experts in prescribing medicines specific to their specialty.

General practitioners are now faced with such a broad spectrum of treatment and medicines that they should treat only what they are fully competent to handle. There is no shame in referring the patient to a qualified specialist. Good doctors always do what is best for the patient.

UNDERSTANDING OFF-LABEL PRESCRIBING

When a new prescription medicine comes to market, it requires FDA approval before it can be promoted for any specific use. This requires evidence-based information that the product has actually been demonstrated to provide the medical benefit that the manufacturer alleges. The research required for FDA approval must also reveal risk and safety information in relation to the patient population being targeted. These matters are covered by evidence-based studies. Before an approval to release the new medicine for public use, the FDA must review all these issues and studies and find there has been an adequate evaluation of benefits and risks.

Once a product is in general use, it isn't unusual for previously unknown side effects and unexpected interactions to be revealed. New uses may also be discovered. A research medication is studied in only a few thousand patients. But, when a drug is released for general use, millions of people will utilize it. As evidence emerges regarding newer uses, a licensed physician is permitted to write prescriptions for these still-unapproved uses, a process known as off-label use. As unexpected adverse reactions or interactions with other drugs are reported, the FDA will notify the physicians and add the information to the product insert pamphlet.

While physicians are permitted to write prescriptions for off-label use, the manufacturer is not permitted to promote already-approved medications for uses that have not passed the oversight mechanisms of the FDA and have not yet been approved for the newly discovered use. When the FDA is satisfied the necessary evidence-based studies have been properly completed, the new use will be added to the product insert. The pharmaceutical company can then promote it.

THE CASE REGARDING NEURONTIN

Obtaining this additional approval is an expensive process. Drug companies have been known to attempt to slip by it. A major example was the Warner-Lambert promotion of Neurontin, an anti-seizure drug for use in neuropathic pain, a symptom I have had only occasional luck relieving with this medication. Some of my colleagues firmly believe it works well for this purpose.

Dr. Sidney Wolfe, author of *Worst Pills, Best Pills*, wrote that Warner-Lambert sponsored the writing of a number of articles that were published in reliable medical journals regarding the off-label benefits of Neurontin in neuralgic pain. Federal investigators determined Warner-Lambert was promoting this use at medical roundtable dinners to which they invited practicing physicians. The federal attorney's office interpreted this as an unapproved indication for Neurontin, fined Warner-Lambert $430 million, and told them to cease this activity. I would not be surprised if Warner-Lambert profits on the prescriptions written for the off-label indication for Neurontin had already exceeded that figure. Neurontin has since been approved for neuralgia, but some studies state this benefit is actually the placebo effect.

CONTROVERSIES REGARDING THE EVALUATION OF CLINICAL TRIALS

Another issue was reported in the *New York Times.*[8] The pharmaceutical industry has apparently funded studies and persuaded well-respected scientists to sign on as co-authors of evidence-based papers regarding these studies, even though those scientists did not participate in the investigations. These reports were then published in peer-reviewed journals. The industry apparently saw to it that papers that supported positive results for their products were published and then promoted by their drug representatives. Papers and reports that failed to support their product or had negative findings were

8 *New York Times*, 17 June 2004.

minimized or not mentioned at all. Although much of the information promoted by the medical literature was probably true, the FDA had not yet approved the drug in question for the use recommended. This may be good for business, but it is certainly not in the spirit of evidence-based medical practice.

In another article about the pharmaceutical industry's clinical trials, the *New York Times* discussed a 1997 federal law that created a government database of clinical trials, ClinicalTrials.gov.[9] It has listed about ten thousand trials since it began operating in 2000. But this law did not require companies or academic institutions to post trial results, nor did it include late-stage Phase III trials or post-approval Phase IV trials. The American Medical Association (AMA), as well as several medical journals such as *Lancet* and *New England Journal of Medicine*, is considering requiring that clinical trials be listed in a comprehensive registry that includes early studies and Phase III and IV results before being accepted for publication.

The *New York Times* reported Merck, the world's second-largest pharmaceutical company, supports the idea of a comprehensive clinical trial registry. However, at that time, none of the other members of the industry was prepared to take a position on the posting of all clinical

9 *New York Times*, 18 June 2004.

trials. Some of the pharmaceutical companies involved in funding research on new drugs were concerned that such a registry might disclose proprietary information to competitors.

The following day, the *New York Times* reporter published an article stating that GlaxoSmithKline, "facing complaints that it selectively disclosed results from pediatric trials of its antidepressant drug Paxil, announced that it planned to create a Web site that would publicly list all clinical trials on its marketed drugs."[10] The *Times* also reported that the attorney general in New York had recently sued GlaxoSmithKline for "misleading doctors by highlighting positive tests of Paxil in depressed youngsters while effectively burying trials with negative findings."

The next day, a firestorm of controversy was on the letters to the editor page and an editorial entitled "For Truth in Drug Reporting."[11] Opinions ranged from the fear on the part of one physician that negative data might be published in lesser journals or not at all to concern that pharmaceutical company financial support would influence how scientists reported negative data and how it could prevent their publication totally. One letter called for disclosure of doctor's compensation that

---

10 *New York Times*, 19 June 2004.

11 "Editorials/Letters," *New York Times*, 20 June 2004.

was itemized for trial design, patient recruitment, and implementation.

The *New York Times* published one more article detailing the issue of publication of clinical trials' results in evidence-based journals.[12] The consensus of editors of several major journals, who the *New York Times* reporter interviewed, was that there indeed should be a registry that would require the listing of all clinical studies. Furthermore, their opinion was that the government should control the registry, not the pharmaceutical industry. The article cited one particular drug, Celexa, an antidepressant that has been approved for use in adults, but has no current approval for use in children. Forest, the distributor in the United States, submitted several papers for publication suggesting Celexa's value as an antidepressant for children, but it never mentioned or referred to articles that had reported negative effects and suicide attempts by children who took the drug. One negative report was in the Danish literature.

The discussion was much more detailed in the *New York Times* article. For those interested in more detail it would be worth looking up an article, "A Medical Journal Quandary: How to Report on Drug Trials."[13]

---

12 *New York Times*, 21 June 2004.

13 *New York Times*, 23 June 2004.

The discussion about Celexa reminded me of the Prozac uproar that Scientology created several years ago. Scientologists reported Prozac, an antidepressant, was causing suicidal and murderous behavior on the part of people who were taking the drug. They claimed they had amassed numerous incidents of this. At the time, several well-known physicians denied this was happening to patients taking Prozac. Most practicing physicians, including myself, discounted Scientology's allegations because most medical scientists do not generally accept Scientology's teachings. I still do not believe in the practice of Scientology, but, in view of the Celexa controversy, maybe there was more than a molecule of truth in what Scientology said about Prozac.[14]

Days after the previous article was published, the *New York Times* wrote that several congressmen were looking at the clinical trials reporting registry issue, possibly promulgating a federal law that would require registration of all clinical trials. Under this law, companies would be required to register a test when it starts and report its results or reason why it was ended. Policymakers said they took such action because of concerns that drug industry sponsorship of such tests was affecting quality. Additionally, medical journals tend to spotlight tests

14 Recent studies have suggested that Prozac did have such risks in children.

with positive findings compared to those with negative or inconclusive results.

The AMA subsequently stated that a centralized clinical trials registry would make it much easier for researchers, physicians, and the general public to access this information. Furthermore, the hope is that easy access to the registry would prevent researchers from duplicating each other's efforts as well as allow physicians to make better treatment decisions. In my view, the patients who might eventually use the new drugs being studied will be safer if a comprehensive clinical drug trial registry is available to clinicians, researchers, and evidence-based medical journals. The journal editors have acknowledged this.

A PERSONAL PROSPECTIVE ABOUT DRUG STUDIES

In my personal medical practice, I have listened to thousands of drug company representatives tout their company's products, but rarely have they ever showed me a single negative article about their own product, even though I knew they existed. I am seldom shown head-to-head studies. Few are done. A head-to-head study compares similar medicines that are in the same drug class and are promoted for the treatment of the same disease process. A well-planned head-to-head study should use equivalent doses of the drugs being compared. The patient population should be as similar as possible. Ideally, there should be a blind crossover period so the patients and doctors are unaware of which medicines are being used in each group.

These studies are rarely done because they usually show very little difference, if any, between medicines in the same drug class. It's not good business for a company to fund head-to-head studies crafted to real evidence-based standards, but it's good medicine.

THE SCIENTIFIC METHOD: THE GOLD STANDARD OF MEDICINE

The scientific method does not accept testimony, impressions, or anecdotes as proof of the effectiveness of a product. Patient testimonials are only a starting point that may suggest a substance or treatment is worthy of investigation. If you listen to your local radio station, especially on Sunday mornings, you will hear people reporting miraculous results obtained by using the vitamin or herb concoction being promoted. Someone calling himself or herself a doctor is often touting the product. He or she is not always a medical doctor, but the same person attests his or her own scientific knowledge and experience has demonstrated the unquestionable value of the product being sold.

WHY THE SCIENTIFIC METHOD IS THE GOLD STANDARD

Valid scientific investigation requires that neither the investigators nor patients know which group is receiving the product being studied and which group is getting the placebo. The identity of the patients and medicines are only revealed when there is a clearly beneficial effect in one group and failure in the others or when the study is totally indecisive.

All medical research is performed on animals until there is reason to believe it is safe to do human trials. In these trials, if one group of patients and not the other group derive a significant benefit, the scientific method requires a crossover be done. The patients are unaware of the crossover. The placebo group of patients starts receiving the medicine that the other group was getting. The other group starts receiving the placebo. The identity of the patients and medicines are only revealed when there is a clearly beneficial effect from one substance and no benefit from the other or when the study is totally indecisive.

In order to maintain objectivity, the doctors and other participating scientists are also unaware of which group is receiving the medicine. This process is known as a double-blind crossover study. As a participant in the Harvard-supervised Physicians' Health Study since it began years ago, I still have no idea if I am taking placebos or the real thing or if there has been a crossover.

Traditionally, human clinical trials have been done at university clinics and hospitals, where the university research staff directly makes requests for human volunteers. The Physicians' Health Study is seeking to analyze the protective effects of certain vitamins. It originally involved four pills. At the onset of the study, we were asked not to attempt to have them analyzed, which, as physicians, we could easily accomplish.

During the next several years, we were told to discard the remaining supply of three of the pills because the research panel concluded the group taking the real pill had demonstrated no benefits over the placebo group. Future shipments came without the pills that had been proved to be of no medical value. On this basis, the fact I had never been informed if I was taking the real pills or placebos or was part of a crossover does not make any difference. The real medications had no discernible benefit or detriment anyway. I am still participating in this research study.

A DANGEROUS TREND

In recent years, community-based physicians have been encouraged to participate in clinical trials on their own patients. I have been concerned about this trend. I know most physicians are motivated to participate for sincerely altruistic reasons, but the remuneration can be very profitable. Unfortunately, there have been cases where personal gain has outstripped altruism.

An incident of this sort, which the news media has documented well, occurred in Los Angeles a few years ago. A physician engaged his patients in a clinical trial that a research-oriented pharmaceutical firm paid for. One of the requirements for the patient to be included in the research panel was that his or her urine specimen had to have certain characteristics. This doctor kept a container of urine with the necessary characteristics in his clinic refrigerator. When a urine sample was required, he submitted a sample from that container in place of the patient's true specimen. One of his employees realized this was unethical behavior and reported his activities to the authorities. It concerns me that such underhanded actions, disguised as scientific research, could escape detection. The approval of new medicines is based on the expectation that the clinical studies have been conducted honorably.

It's understandable that well-meaning physicians may have doubts or ambivalence about participating in clinical trials on their own patients or even referring them for this purpose. Important issues must be considered. The Los Angeles County Medical Association/Bar Association Joint Committee on Biomedical Ethics developed guidelines for physicians who plan to be involved in human clinical trials.[15]

Among the issues discussed in the guidelines are informed consent and benefits to the patient, if any.

---

15 Los Angeles County Medical Association, "Participation in Clinical Drug or Device Trials: Guidelines for the Community Physician," 2002.

The guidelines also outline what the referring physician should learn about the clinical trial program being promoted to them before they agree to participate. A copy of these guidelines is available from the Los Angeles County Medical Association for those interested in reading the actual text.

LEARNING TO APPRECIATE THE SCIENTIFIC METHOD

As an undergraduate student, I was taught to use the scientific approach when evaluating evidence. I recall the laboratory sessions where each student was expected to perform certain laboratory procedures. No matter how careful the students were, the results often came out different than expected. Utilizing the scientific method, the student is encouraged to retrace the steps of the experiment in an effort to find out what went wrong.

Out of this experience comes the understanding that results are not always what's expected, no matter how carefully the process was performed. In medical practice, when a patient's test result seems to be inconsistent with the suspected disease process, the doctor will sometimes repeat the test in order to be certain the laboratory didn't make an error. In my own practice, if I question the results, I sometimes repeat the test at a different laboratory so I can compare them. I only do that when

I am truly perplexed about an important lab result because insurance companies often aren't willing to pay for redundant tests.

In laboratory classes at college, grades usually depended on the accuracy of the results of the test being done. After all, we were supposed to be learning to do reliable laboratory work. Grades were important to undergraduate students because admission to graduate school or medical school was based on them. Some of the students turned in what they knew to be the correct results in order to get a good grade, even if their results were incorrect. But a true scientist never "dry labs" anything. If a result comes out different than expected, so be it. A true scientist either accepts the result or does it over again while trying to avoid prior errors. That's the scientific method. Scientific experiments, by definition, are reproducible. Everybody doing an experiment correctly will get the same result.

A while ago, some scientists claimed they had achieved cold fusion. If that was true, it could revolutionize the energy production industry. To this day, no other lab has been able to reproduce the results of the experiment. The ability to reproduce results is how science proves facts. Until that's done, cold fusion will be regarded as a process that has not yet been accomplished. As a scientist and a physician, I rely upon the ethics and honesty of evidence-based medicine. There is absolutely no place for dishonesty and misdirection in science and medicine.

ETHICS, HONESTY, AND MEDICINE

An article in the *Wall Street Journal* entitled "Science Breaks Down When Cheaters Think They Won't Be Caught" disturbed me. The author contends there will always be cheaters and believes peer-reviewed journals and rules of scientific collaboration keep failing us. She goes on to cite numerous examples of cheating and falsification of data by well-known scientists.

That wasn't the only time I have read about falsification of data published in peer-reviewed journals. As stated earlier, a prominent pharmaceutical company was disappointed with the sales of a new medicine it manufactured. To promote the medication to doctors, it paid physicians who were not involved in the research to sign on to the journal articles as if they were involved. The articles were then published so the manufacturer could establish a new use for the medication and boost prescription sales. The FDA had not yet approved those new uses. The company paid a significant fine for promoting their drug for a use not yet approved. I suspect it was worth it to them.

I was appalled by reports that some manufacturers have withheld information about adverse reactions because that information could hurt sales. I wrote a number of letters to the editorial pages of major newspapers, expressing my concern for patient safety when physicians prescribe medications that might cause serious adverse reactions about which they were not warned. Some of those medicines were subsequently taken off the market because of journalistic diligence that publicized the information and the FDA's response to those facts.

Corporate greed and dishonesty and its effect on the stock market are well-known to investors. These practices affect our fiscal health, which is bad enough, but scientific and medical dishonesty affects our physical well-being. And that is intolerable.

WHY YOU SHOULD READ THE PACKAGE INSERT

The FDA requires a package insert accompany every package of prescription medicine shipped from a pharmaceutical manufacturing facility. Also known as the product brochure, this literature contains detailed descriptive information about the medicine that the package contains.

Not only does this information sheet come with every unopened container of medicine received by the retail pharmacy, but packages of samples distributed to physicians also contain this information. Furthermore, every advertisement that appears in the professional medical journals, as well the consumer publications, has this information printed next to the ad. The purpose is to provide educational reference material to the retail pharmacist, prescribing physician, and consumer, if they choose to read it.

CONFUSION, COMPLAINTS, AND SOLUTIONS

In recent times, the format of this information has been questioned. Some pharmaceutical industry spokespersons disclaim responsibility. They have blamed some adverse reactions and even deaths that were attributed to certain newly marketed medicines on physician failure to adequately read the warnings and contraindications printed in the product brochures.

The response to this accusation is that the product brochure is too confusing. A series of articles on the subject appeared in newspapers. One journalist pointed out that the first information about adverse reactions often missed by the prescribing doctors was over two hundred lines into the document. Also, the material was not organized in a way that permitted easy access to and emphasis on vital prescribing information.

At the time of this controversy, I examined a number of contemporary and typical FDA drug information inserts. In each, the opening paragraphs, "Description," discussed the chemistry and class (family) and chemical structure of the active ingredient. The second section, "Clinical Pharmacology," discussed the pharmacodynamics and metabolism of the product (how it works in the body). Depending on the product, this section might discuss such matters as:

- Absorption
- Distribution in the body, most effective and safe as formulated
- Mode of excretion

- Effects on special populations such as geriatric, pediatric, and people who could be adversely affected because of certain pathological conditions such as seizure and other disorders

Animal studies are reported as well as information on propensities such as cancer genesis and effects on pregnant animals and their fetuses. Clinical studies often follow and may include drug-drug interreactions. The all-important warnings section follows. This paragraph might be printed in all capitals or boldface or, in extreme cases, a black enclosure (the infamous black box). A separate paragraph will be devoted to adverse reactions. Indications and usage would usually appear here. Dosage and administration advice follows this information.

The brochure could be as short as a standard-sized, two-sided sheet, fully printed in small print. Or it could be as long as a several-page booklet with much more information. The criticism is that the product brochure is so detailed that it obscures the descriptions of warnings, adverse reactions, and dosage information needed by the doctor prescribing the drug.

Medicines are accompanied by a pamphlet for the patient to read, usually to describe how to take the medicine and any special warnings about its use. In the case of birth control pills, for example, smoking is contraindicated, though that warning too often goes unheeded.

THE NEW FORMAT MAKES FINDING INFORMATION EASIER

On January 14, 2006, the FDA announced a new prescription drug brochure format that was designed to improve patient safety. It was the first major revision in more than twenty-five years. The new format requires a summary of the most important information about the product, and it was to be prominently displayed at the top of the first page of the brochure. It also includes:

- A highlights section that provides the most important information about benefits and risks
- A patient counseling information section to help doctors advise about uses, limitations, and risks
- A table of contents for easy reference
- The date of the initial product approval

The FDA believes this will be a more user-friendly format for the physician and pharmacist without losing any of the information that the prescriber may consider important. As new information regarding usage comes to the FDA, it may be included in revisions of the product brochure. However, such new uses must be supported by studies done at reliable institutions via clinical trials and evidence-based reports in the medical literature.

As this is written, some of the newly formatted package inserts have already been published. Some of the older medicine packages still contain the unrevised insert, but the updated information is available from other sources.

The FDA encourages physicians to report any untoward effects they may become aware of. The forms for reporting adverse reaction are readily available to doctors. If a pattern seems to arise from these reports, the FDA may send an alert to practicing physicians describing the new information and then subsequently add it to later versions of the product brochure. If a serious risk of harm to patients emerges, the FDA may require the manufacturer to withdraw the product from the marketplace.

In my long career as a physician, I have occasionally sent adverse effect reports (FDA Med Watch Form 3500) to the FDA. Not only have I seen a number of drugs removed from the marketplace, but I have happily seen numerous revisions and improvements in the product brochures.

HOW MEDICINES WORK

Thanks to cell biologists, we are learning how the body works. That information has led to the development of many worthwhile medicines.

Medicines augment useful biological functions and inhibit harmful ones. It is not unusual for the pharmaceutical industry to describe a class of drugs by what it does. The researchers endeavor to develop a substance that has a maximum of desirable effects with a minimum of side effects. No matter how carefully this goal is pursued, there are no medicines without side effects to someone. Some side effects are common to the class of drugs to which the substance in question belongs. But each substance may have unique effects that none other in the class share.

HOW THE BODY CHEMISTRY USES MEDICINES

Sometimes, patients who are taking several medicines at a time ask how each drug knows where to go. I assure them that cell biology makes it possible for each medicine to find its way. But there are exceptions to that rule. If two drugs use the same biological pathway to do their work, they may interfere with each other.

Cells have a number of ways to perform the function for which they are intended. As a physician, I am not expected to know them all, but it is critical to know the important ones. Three of the major processes by which cells function are known as channels, converting enzymes, and receptor sites. The functional process is often designated by the operating enzyme, a letter, and a number.

- The channel is the physiological pathway that takes a body chemical or a medicine to the site where it will function.
- The converting enzymes are biological agents that are able to change a substance from one form into another. To work as a detoxifying agent, the converting enzyme changes an active substance into a less active or inactive form. Converting enzymes also function to turn inactive precursors into active forms. An example of this bodily function is the natural conversion of angiotensin I into angiotensin II. Angiotensin II acts on the arteries to constrict them, thus raising the blood pressure. This is an important function, as there are times when the body needs a rise in blood pressure to perform certain activities. Angiotensin II can also be

responsible for persistent and undesirable high blood pressure, so the pharmaceutical industry developed angiotensin enzyme blockers. They prevent angiotensin I from becoming the blood pressure-raising angiotensin II. These drugs, Angiotensin-Converting Enzyme (ACE) inhibitors, are also widely used in heart failure patients and diabetics.

- The operating enzyme is the body substance that will convert the medicine or body chemical into an active or detoxified form.
- The letter or number designates which channel and/or body substance is participating in the process. Among the best known are the cytochrome P450 oxidase channels, which are found in the liver cells. They function as detoxifying channels and keep potentially dangerous substances from harming the body.

WHY THE DOCTOR MUST UNDERSTAND THE BODY'S CHEMISTRY

Physicians must know which of the medicines they are prescribing are detoxified via one of these mechanisms. Many substances and medicines utilize this process. At times, a channel or enzyme becomes so overutilized that it can't keep up with the load. In those circumstances, a medicine could accumulate to a toxic level in the body because the biological mechanisms are unable to accommodate it. An example of this is the once-common simultaneous use of the bronchodialator theophylline and antibiotic erythromycin.

Although physicians usually got away with the joint use of these two medicines, there was concern that the toxic effects of excessive levels of theophylline could cause undesireable tachycardia (fast heart rate). This particular combination of medicines are now rarely used at the same time.

THE RECEPTOR SITE

Another frequently utilized method of action in the body is the receptor site. I am reminded of *Dr. Ehrlich's Magic Bullet*, a movie I saw as a youngster. That movie was one of the influences that led me into the study of the sciences. In that movie (and allegedly in history), Dr. Ehrlich did six hundred and six chemical trials until he found a drug that arrested syphilis. That drug was Salvarsan (606), an arsenic derivative. Ehrlich hypothesized this chemical had a molecular shape that keyed into a receptor site on the syphilis germ and resulted in its death, thus controlling the disease. Receptor sites are widely hypothesized in many situations.

Another example is the action of insulin in the human body. Diabetes is a disease in which insulin fails to function properly to control blood glucose levels. Normal blood glucose levels vary from between sixty and one hundred forty (measured in milligrams per one hundred cubic centimeters of blood). The maximum blood glucose level for a fasting patient was recently reduced to one hundred twenty-six, a standard that added more than a million people to the group of individuals at risk for diabetes.[16] A level above one hundred sixty at any time is considered borderline diabetes. Above two hundred is considered diabetes that is not well-controlled.[17]

Although there are several causes of diabetes, it is usually thought of as taking two forms. They were formerly called juvenile and maturity onset diabetes. They are also known as type I and type II diabetes. I prefer the terminology insulin-dependent and non-insulin-dependent diabetes because it more accurately describes the way the two categories of the disease are usually treated.

Insulin-dependent diabetes is characterized by inadequate amounts of insulin, so the patient must take additional insulin to make up the needed difference. Non-insulin-dependent diabetics have more than enough insulin, but many of the patient's insulin receptor sites

16 Authorities are considering lowering the level even further.

17 These numbers were regarded as accurate when I wrote this. I tell my patients that the standards in medical practice "change every Tuesday and Thursday and sometimes on Wednesday."

aren't functioning so blood glucose levels are not well controlled and the levels get too high.

In response to the receptor site issue, the pharmaceutical industry has produced diabetes-controlling medications that make insulin receptor sites more sensitive to insulin. An excess of insulin subjects a diabetic patient to the risk of hypoglycemia (low blood sugar). Insulin-dependent diabetics are always at risk of developing hypoglycemia, especially if they don't have something to eat proximate to injecting their insulin.

When I first started my medical practice, urine glucose levels were the usual way to check how well the patient was controlling his or her diabetes. The urine sample was put into a test tube, along with a testing solution, and heated over a gas flame. A color change revealed the presence of glucose. That test was helpful, but not very accurate. The doctor could obtain a blood glucose with a small quantity of blood obtained by a painful lancet puncture. This was usually sent to a laboratory for a more accurate blood glucose reading.

Today's testing science has made the blood glucose test the standard and very accurate. The patient is now able to obtain a tiny quantity of blood painlessly. A small battery-operated meter immediately flashes the accurate blood glucose level on its screen. In any circumstances, diabetes is always a balancing act. Some patients never seem to get their diabetes under control.

Although there are many other mechanisms of drug action, these simplistic examples will provide some concept of how each medicine that the patient is taking knows where to go to do its work and one of the many ways they sometimes interfere with each other's action.

EXPIRATION, INTERACTION, AND DURATION

The question of when a medicine gets too old to use safely has always been a perplexing one for the public as well as doctors. How can a medicine be perfectly safe the day before its expiration date and useless the day after? Rather than take the risk of ingesting a useless or even harmful substance, many medicines have been discarded when they reaches their expiration dates, even though they were actually still safe and effective. At one lecture I attended, I heard a pharmacologist from the local medical school claim that some medicinal substances would still be effective after being found buried in the Pharaoh's tomb.

There are many ways the safety and efficacy of some medicines can be harmful. Some medicines are packed with a desiccant that protects them from moisture that might cause deterioration. Medicines that are subject to damage by light must be stored in opaque or lightproof containers. Heat or freezing can damage some products. Many medicines may deteriorate because of oxidation or aging. Obviously, both expiration dates and the way the medication is stored have a role and should be obeyed.

EXPIRATION DATES

In recent years, several issues have caused the regulatory agencies to rethink expiration dates. One is the unnecessary waste of costly, still-effective medicines by patients who can ill afford to buy a fresh supply. Second, the possibility of events such as an epidemic, for example the flu, or the current ongoing fear of bioterrorism validate the need to have a national stockpile of certain vital drugs that could be immediately accessed. We hope the need for those stockpiled drugs never arises, but our society must be prepared for any event.

The Shelf Life Extension Program, a joint effort between the FDA and Department of Defense, has addressed the issue. The FDA is now evaluating shelf lives of many important and expensive medicines in order to extend the safe and effective expiration date. It could save medicine users millions of dollars.

I recall a physician colleague whom I knew years ago. Every year, he returned to his native South American country, using his vacation time to work at a free clinic. Before he left the United States, he'd have his physician friends save all of their expired medicine samples to take with him to his free clinic, where they were distributed to the needy patients. According to him, they were just as effective as the drugs labeled with a date that had not yet expired.

Some drugs actually reveal when they are past their expiration date, for example, by color change or odor. These changes may reduce efficacy, but not always. Aspirin, for example, takes on a vinegary odor when it ages, although it is still effective. Adrenalin changes from colorless to pink when it ages. If used, it may cause hallucinations. So I discard it rather than expose my patients to that possibility. The lesson is that, if a medication is beyond its expiration date, ask your doctor for advice.

DRUG INTERACTIONS

When more than one medicine is prescribed for a patient, the doctor must consider possible interactions between them. This is often no easy task. When the benefits of multiple drug therapy clearly outweigh the risks, it is important to cautiously use the combination of drugs even though they could have potential interactions. The patient should be warned of that possibility and told to call for advice should an unexpected effect occur.

The computer information age has helped to some extent. Now, computer programs oversee prescriptions and call the pharmacist's attention to possible interactions when several prescriptions for medicines are filled at the same time. However, prescriptions are not always filled at the same time or in the same pharmacy. Furthermore, knowledge of interactions between drugs, food, and other substances may be unknown until incidents are reported and the FDA adds information to the product brochure.

A computer cannot always identify another problem, the reaction between the medicine being prescribed and what the patient is doing, drinking, or eating. For example, a person shouldn't drive after taking a medicine that can cause sedation. So he or she should be made aware of that possibility. Some foods may either delay or enhance the absorption of certain medicines. A good example is the binding of some antibiotics to milk products. This can actually keep some types of antibiotics from being absorbed by the gastrointestinal tract. When such interactions are known to exist, the dispensing pharmacist will usually print an appropriate warning on the receptacle's label.

Another common food that interferes with the absorption of some medicines is grapefruit. If a frequent user of grapefruit or grapefruit juice is required to take medicine in the same time frame, the pharmacist or doctor should be consulted regarding the compatibility of the two. If there is the possibility of interference with the absorption, the patient should avoid ingesting grapefruit at the same time he takes the medicine.

One of the strangest administration instructions is for the family of osteoporosis-correcting medications, such as Fosamax, Actonel, and Boniva. The patient is instructed that these medicines must be taken with a full glass of plain water at least a half hour before food, other beverage, or medicine. After the medicine is swallowed, the patient must remain in an upright position for a half hour before eating. Food interferes with absorption of this family of medicines. The upright position minimizes regurgitation of the medicine back into the esophagus, where it could cause irritation or even ulceration. Therefore, the reason for the detailed instructions about how to take these medicines.

MOST MEDICINES TAKE TIME TO COMPLETE THE TREATMENT

A frequent problem that physicians have with patients is getting them to use their medication for the period of time prescribed. Patients often feel better shortly after beginning the treatment, and the sense of well-being convinces them that their affliction has been cured. This is especially true of infections that require antibiotics. The doctor is aware that too short a course of antibiotics sometimes leads to a relapse of the infection and may even lead to the emergence of an antibiotic-resistant strain of the infecting organism. Too long a course is wasteful and could result in a secondary infection by an organism that is not responsive to the antibiotic being used.

THE PROBLEM OF UNRESPONSIVE SECONDARY INFECTION

An example of this is when an antibiotic kills off the bowel's natural E. coli bacteria population. The patient may experience an overgrowth of Clostridium difficile, a bacteria that is present in low count in the bowels of many people. The bowel's normal E. coli population keeps the C. difficile growth in check. The drop in E. coli concentration may allow the Clostridium difficile to multiply unopposed. Clostridium difficile is so named because it is difficult to kill with our usual antibiotics. When it's able to grow without opposition, it produces a toxin that causes copious diarrhea, an illness known as pseudomembranous colitis. It requires the use of special antibiotics such as Flagyl and vancomycin to suppress the Clostridium difficile and special resins to absorb the toxin it produces.

Most antibiotics obliterate the infection being treated in seven to ten days, but antibiotics used in diseases such as tuberculosis may require six months to a year of treatment. Some antibiotics, such as Azithromax, need only to be taken for three to five days. There's now also a one-day (single) dose. Azithromax has been demonstrated to continue its action for up to ten days.

Recent studies have suggested that a five-day course of an effective antibiotic may be sufficient for hospitalized patients with antibiotic-sensitive pneumonia. This is believed to minimize the emergence of resistant hospital infections. Medicines such as bronchodilators and painkillers can be stopped as soon as the symptoms subside.

MEDICINES FOR CHRONIC CONDITIONS

Medications used for chronic conditions, such as high blood pressure, heart disease, diabetes, and so forth, will often be needed for lifelong duration. Medication controls these conditions, but does not cure them. Stopping the medicine allows the condition to flare up again. Some of these diseases require multiple, lifelong drugs to lengthen life span in patients who take them. Heart disease is best controlled by taking several drugs from different categories for the rest of the patient's life.

Research studies have shown that this tactic lengthens life span in patients who take such drug combinations when compared to the control group of patients who aren't taking such a combination. Combinations are said to be cardioprotective. Polypharmacy (use of multiple medications) is discouraged where there it not a definite benefit to be achieved. Every medicine has risks!

Some medicines have a relatively short duration of action. In as little as a few hours, they must be taken again. Some are as often as every four hours. The effect of drugs like nitroglycerine lasts only minutes. The directions suggest the patient should repeat the dose in five minutes if there has been no relief of chest pain after the first dose.

The problem of short-acting medicines is under treatment because of missed (forgotten) doses. The pharmaceutical industry has largely solved this problem by developing various methods of slowing the medicine's rate of release or lengthening its duration of action.

Although this process has generally been well accepted and is highly successful, there are drawbacks. If a person becomes allergic to the drug or overreacts to the ingredients for any reason, the long-action effect may prolong the adverse reactions.

SPLITTING OR BREAKING PILLS

Splitting and breaking pills is a popular way to save money on medicine because the pricing structure of many medicines is often less than double for a pill that is twice as strong. The drug industry even encourages this in some cases. But if a prescribed medicine pill is designated as long acting or is marketed as having extended release, it's wise not to split or break it unless the manufacturer indicates that breaking the pill will not interrupt its long-acting feature.

Some medicines have an enteric coating that doesn't increase the duration of the action, but it does prevent the ingredients from being released until after the pill leaves the stomach. This is usually done because the medicine that is produced with an enteric coating is known to cause irritation of the esophagus and stomach. Breaking the pill destroys this protective barrier.

SIDE EFFECTS AND ALLERGIC REACTIONS: IT'S SOMETIMES HARD TO TELL THE DIFFERENCE

Every prescription medicine has side effects that somebody will get. Some side effects are so common that most persons who take the drug will experience them. Others are so rare that only an occasional user will report having them. It is not the purpose of this book to enumerate the adverse reactions of every class of medicines. The FDA has done that very well in each medicine's product brochure. My purpose is to make the public aware that the risk-versus-benefit issue exists with everything we do, but especially with medicines.

SIDE EFFECTS AND ALLERGIC REACTIONS ARE NOT THE SAME

Allergic reactions are common, but an adverse reaction is not truly a side effect. An allergic reaction is a specific reaction to a substance that a person has been previously exposed and sensitized to. Before prescribing medicines known to cause allergic reactions, it is important to ask the patient if he or she has ever reacted to that family of medicines in the past. For instance, if I'm planning to prescribe Amoxil, a penicillin derivative, I would ask if he or she ever had a reaction to the penicillin family of medicines.

Once, a teenager was brought into my office with an infected throat and high fever. Her graduation from high school was only a few days away, and she didn't want to miss it. She had what I was certain was Strep throat, which is usually treated with ten days of penicillin. She told me she was allergic to penicillin. It had once caused her to break out in a rash. I offered the next most common choice at the time, erythromycin, but she complained that erythromycin had caused her to become nauseated before. We settled on Declomycin, a form of tetracycline that was very popular in those days.

Within a few days, she was fine and able to attend the graduation ceremony. The next morning, her mother called and told me that her daughter must be allergic to the Declomycin because she had broken out in a rash. She wouldn't be able to finish the necessary ten-day course of medicine. The specific rash did not sound typical of an antibiotic allergic reaction, so I asked them to come to the office to let me see it. It was indeed atypical. It spared her face and lower limbs and consisted of comma-shaped red spots on her chest, abdomen, and thighs. She was wearing a bra and panties, and the rash also failed to appear on those covered areas.

I asked what she had worn to the graduation. It had been a typical sunny San Fernando Valley summer day so the graduation was held outdoors. She wore a new lace dress, purchased specifically for the occasion. That was the answer I was seeking. She wasn't allergic to the Declomycin. She had experienced a side effect of that class of antibiotics. The tetracycline family of medicines is known to increase sensitivity to the sun. I usually warn patients not to go to the beach, where they could experience a severe sunburn with a very brief exposure when taking this medicine.

She hadn't worn a petticoat under the fine lace fabric of her dress. She had put a protective suntan lotion on the normally exposed skin surfaces of the face, arms, and legs. The ultraviolet light-sensitizing Declomycin had caused the sun to print the pattern of her lace dress on the usually unexposed, ultraviolet-sensitive areas of her body. Problem solved! This was not an allergic reaction. It was a side effect of this family of medicines. She could finish the ten-day course of antibiotic. She just had to stay out of the sun.

Side effects are often a nuisance that may have to be tolerated if the medicine is important enough to continue using. An oncologist doesn't stop essential chemotherapy in a cancer patient just because it causes the patient's hair to fall out. The benefit achieved is greater than the undesirable effects of the medicine.

A side effect sometimes becomes the main reason for taking the medicine. A well-known antihistamine has the side effect of drowsiness. This is a common side effect of many antihistamines, and it has prompted the development of a whole new family of antihistamines, which are probably no better than the old standbys, Benadryl and chlorpheniramine, but the newer antihistamines cause less drowsiness. Because of the drowsiness induced by these drugs, doctors usually advise that patients taking Benadryl or chlorpheniramine should not drive or operate dangerous equipment. However, the side effect of drowsiness can lead to their use to induce sleep without the habit-forming risk of a sleeping pill.

THE BENEFITS OF A MEDICATION ARE SOMETIMES WORTH THE RISKS

True allergies are not side effects. The allergy may take the form of a rash, hives, generalized itching, nasal congestion, asthmatic respirations, and so forth. An allergic person can even die from an anaphylactic reaction. This is also known as anaphylactic shock. It is manifested by immediate respiratory distress and is followed by vascular collapse (shock). The prompt administration of adrenalin or cortisone may be required to save a life.

Patients don't always relate adverse experiences with the medicines they take. I could fill volumes with stories about patients who reported symptoms they were not aware were being caused by the medicine they were taking. Of these numerous cases of unrecognized adverse reactions, I'm reminded of several from my own medical practice. They taught me object lessons about the inevitability of side effects, and they are worth repeating.

An elderly woman became my patient after she had recovered from a serious infection for which she had spent some weeks in the hospital.

While doing her initial examination, I found she was deaf. I had to obtain all her history from the daughter. I was told that, although she had been somewhat hard of hearing prior to her hospitalization, she had become stone-deaf during the recent illness. The daughter attributed the increased loss of hearing to the intensity of the infection. The hospital doctors had told her it was resistant to most of the antibiotics and had almost caused her mother's death.

I felt it was important I know the details of her mother's hospitalization. A review of the hospital's records revealed the patient did indeed have an infection, which was highly resistant to many antibiotics. In order to save her life, the hospital doctors had to use some of the most powerful antibiotics available at the time. The antibiotic, to which the infection was susceptible, undoubtedly saved her life, but I was aware that one of its side effects was damage to the auditory nerve. That antibiotic probably completed her deafness, but the control of the infection was paramount, and the risk had to be taken.

The risk of dangerous side effects doesn't always have to be taken. My cousin's mother-in-law died from aplastic anemia (a condition where the patient's body stops making new blood cells) caused by a then widely used antibiotic, Chloromycetin. A less powerful antibiotic with fewer risks could easily have treated her infection. If her infection proved to be viral, she may not have had to take an antibiotic at all. Chloromycetin, a wonderfully effective antibiotic, is still available, but now it is infrequently used because of that dangerous side effect. Fortunately, other effective antibiotics are usually available to use in its place.

ACCUTANE

Accutane, another prescription medication, has such significant adverse reactions that the manufacturer has voluntarily restricted its use. Accutane is used to treat the most severe forms of acne with great success.

Unfortunately, it has one major defect and several lesser side effects. It causes birth defects in the fetuses of pregnant women who use it. It can also cause liver, lipid, and pancreatic malfunction. There have been reports of depression, psychosis, suicide attempts, and even successful suicide in patients. Birth defects are a proven risk of Accutane. People who suffer from severe acne might also be depressed by their affliction, even to the extent of thoughts of suicide unrelated to the Accutane itself. The treating physician must be aware that these side effects may occur in the patient under treatment and be prepared to deal with them.

The manufacturer requires all women of childbearing age be tested for pregnancy before it can be prescribed. They also suggest that certain liver, pancreas, and lipid tests be done before the start of treatment and periodically after the treatment is started. I have chosen to no longer prescribe it for females of childbearing age, although I have successfully done so in the past. In my view, the cosmetic benefits may be outweighed by the risks entailed. These facts must be seriously discussed with every patient before prescribing Accutane.[18]

Many effective ways of treating acne entail fewer risks than those attributed to Accutane, although probably none of those treatments is as effective as Accutane.

18 Google the internet for details about the drug Accutane.

Unfortunately, people are willing to undergo substantial suffering and take significant risk to achieve what they view as desirable cosmetic benefits.

A SIDE EFFECT NOT PREVIOUS DESCRIBED

Pain is another malady that drives people to take risks. I have treated many patients with headaches. I have had to refer some to a headache clinic, but my theme that all medicines are poison reminds me of one patient in particular, who chose what she thought was the less risky way of controlling her pain. She experienced an adverse effect that nobody knew existed. She suffered from headaches for most of her life and found Empirin compound, an OTC medicine, was as good as anything she had taken before. It was not known to be addicting. It was certainly less expensive and, in her opinion, safer than a prescription medicine. At the time she started taking it, most doctors, including myself, would have agreed that it had all of the advantages she ascribed to it.

One day, she became quite ill, so I hospitalized her. Studies showed she was suffering from renal (kidney) failure. About the time she became ill, an Australian physician published a medical journal paper reporting that high doses of phenacetin had been found to cause renal failure. I realized Empirin compound contained phenacetin as one of its ingredients. My patient had been taking it in high doses for years.

I called a nephrologist, who confirmed the diagnosis and advised my patient to stop using phenacetin. Even though she stopped taking it, the damage was done. Eventually, she had to have dialysis treatments to control her uremia. I subsequently lost contact with her. I do not know if she ever received a kidney transplant.

It was later reported that all analgesics of the phenacetin type could cause kidney damage. Phenacetin was taken off the market. Many other analgesics can potentially cause kidney damage if used excessively. Among those analgesics are the NSAIDs, of which there are many, including Motrin, Advil, and ibuprofen, to name a few. They are available as OTC or prescription. They can be generic or have a name brand. They can all cause kidney disease and liver problems if not used carefully. Patients who use these medications regularly should be tested for kidney and liver function.

SIDE EFFECTS AS BENEFITS

Some years ago, a new antihypertensive drug named Rogaine arrived on the prescription market. It wasn't a very profitable blood pressure-lowering medicine, but it was found to have a prominent side effect, which eventually created an entirely new market for the substance. It caused unexpected hair growth in the people who used it as an antihypertensive drug. The research team who studied this side effect found that, when provided as a lotion or solution that could be applied to areas of thinning hair or bald spots, it would promote hair growth and have a desirable cosmetic effect. What was formerly an adverse reaction became the product's major use. This litany has repeated itself numerous times, although usually less dramatically than the Rogaine story.

BURDENS AND BENEFITS

Diuretics were originally developed to remove excess fluid from the body. Most diuretics tend to cause the body to lose potassium, a troublesome side effect that often requires corrective measures. But that side effect can be useful for patients who have accumulated excessive blood levels of potassium. Excessive accumulation of potassium can be very detrimental, even to the extent of causing cardiac standstill and death, so limiting the excessive accumulation of potassium can be vitally important. The converse (too low of a potassium level) causes profound weakness and can cause cardiac rhythm disorders.

The other side effect of diuretics, the removal of sodium from the body, was another benefit that originally brought diuretics to the marketplace. This effect can benefit fluid retention syndromes, such as edema and heart failure. The removal of sodium is also useful in controlling high blood pressure. Hypertension can be made worse by eating too much salty food. Table salt is chemically known as sodium chloride. Doctors usually prescribe a low-sodium diet for hypertensive patients. The old saying, "One man's meat is another man's poison," applies here. Benefits can be burdens; burdens can be benefits.

WE SOMETIMES MUST BE WILLING TO ACCEPT SIDE EFFECTS

My patients know that all medicines have side effects for some people because I show them the adverse reactions section of the FDA product brochure that describes what they are and the frequency of their occurrence. If the benefits outweigh the risks, then I prescribe the indicated medication. They must be willing to accept some mild side effects, such as dry mouth or drowsiness. If the benefit is important enough, they must be willing to accept even more bothersome effects such as urinary frequency and diarrhea. I have personally experienced these side effects from medicines that were prescribed to me. The side effects were well worth enduring in exchange for the benefits I derived.

When I was in heart failure after experiencing a myocardial infarction (heart attack), I was given a potent diuretic that drained the excess fluid out of my body. As the result of this necessary treatment with a diuretic, I subsequently had a very painful attack of gout. My doctor prescribed colchicine, an ancient treatment for gout. It is still one of the safest and most effective remedies for this disease, but it can cause severe diarrhea. When it is prescribed, the patient is told to use it until the gout attack subsides or until diarrhea occurs. Then the patient is to stop.

Some side effects are unacceptable. I expect the patient or family to call me if a rash, bleeding, or unanticipated pain or breathing difficulty occurs or if the patient experiences a sudden change of mental status or loss of consciousness. When the risks outweigh the benefits, the medicine must be stopped or changed. If necessary, a medication to treat the side effect must be prescribed. With many medicines, especially those taken for the long term, certain organs can be adversely affected and must be tested periodically. Some medications can adversely affect the liver, kidneys, or blood count. To be certain that such undesirable effects haven't occurred, it's best to follow the patient with blood tests and/or urinalysis. Where no treatment is required, I do nothing!

MEDICINES AND TREATMENTS MUST BE THOROUGHLY TESTED

I'd scarcely become a family physician in 1961 when I found out how dangerous prescribing can be if a doctor doesn't have a thorough knowledge of the medicine and its adverse reactions. As a new doctor, I wasn't very busy so I spent my free time reading journals. In those days, the *Journal of the American Medical Association* had a section with English abstracts of articles translated from foreign journals. It still does today.

I noted with interest an article from Germany expressing concern about a new drug I'd never heard of before called thalidomide. It was suspected to be causing limb deformities (phocomelia) in the newborns of women who took it during their pregnancy. A few weeks later, a drug company representative called me and offered to supply me with a new sedative that the FDA had not fully released for marketing. It was thalidomide. I was surprised he was unaware of the reports from Europe. Although it was permissible in those days for a licensed physician to participate in pre-marketing clinical trials, I declined the samples that were being offered to me.

A few months later, I read the FDA was not going to allow the release of thalidomide in the United States because pre-marketing clinical trials had revealed limb birth defects in the offspring of pregnant women who had used it.

I was very proud of the FDA for avoiding a possible disaster. In the years that followed, I saw several cases of phocomelia. This impressed on me the necessity of reading the warnings and adverse reactions as well as interactions of all medicines I prescribe. It also gave me a subsequent lifelong need to avoid any product that was not subjected to thorough animal and human clinical evaluation. Many OTC products have never had the advantage of this sort of scrutiny.

I firmly believe all substances for which there are claims of health or medical treatment benefits should be subjected to studies to determine if these benefits really exist and, if they do, what risks and burdens are also possible. Medical history has many examples of substances and treatments that were proved to be of true value and were eventually adopted as part of traditional medical care, but there were also some disasters.

This essay illustrates why the practice of medicine is sometimes called an art. The physician's skill must not only make an accurate diagnosis, but also prescribe a treatment that cures the patient with the least amount of harm and discomfort. The physician must consider the risk of an allergic reaction or side effects and, if one of these should occur, how to deal with it in the most effective and expedient way.

THE ROLE OF SANITATION IN DISEASE PREVENTION

I'm reminded of Ignatz Phillipp Semmelweis, who was ridiculed when he insisted that hand washing was an important way to prevent puerperal fever, a form of febrile sepsis that often infected mothers after childbirth in his day. It was subsequently demonstrated that Semmelweis was right. Antisepsis and aseptic technique has become a standard of medicine since then.

The reference to Dr. Semmelweis' historic work reminds me of the saying, "what goes around, comes around." As previously pointed out, the United States is currently experiencing a dramatic incidence of hospital-acquired infections. It was observed that caregivers, including nurses and doctors, were not washing their hands between patient contacts. Now every hospital has hand disinfection units at locations near each patient room. Doctors and all hospital personnel are required to use them.

The importance of the contact transfer of infection was dramatically brought to my attention during a recent vacation on a large cruise ship. The cruise ship industry has been plagued by intestinal infections among its guests. The outbreaks are characterized by diarrhea and/or nausea and vomiting. The Public Health Service believes the Norwalk virus (norovirus infection) causes this illness. An outbreak on my vacation cruise prompted the captain to require over one hundred infected people to be isolated in their cabins. The rest of us were not permitted to touch any food or serving utensil. Gloved crewmembers (using calipers) served us everything. Hand disinfectant dispensers were everywhere, and we were required to use them before entering the dining areas. Even the handrails throughout the ship were disinfected regularly. All of this inconvenience paid off. In five days, the epidemic was controlled, and the quarantine was ended.

Several years since our own experience with the Norwalk virus shipboard outbreak, the Norwalk virus outbreaks still plague the cruise ships, despite all of the hand disinfection being used. I have seen an increase of gastroenteritis in long-term nursing facilities. They are now also encouraging the use of hand disinfectants.

MY OWN EXPERIENCE

As a former consulting sanitation inspector with the California State Public Health Department, I investigated a similar, but much more serious, sanitation-related outbreak. I was assigned to find out why a facility that housed mentally deficient children was having hepatitis outbreaks. The facility consisted of several ward units completely isolated from each other. Some of the wards were infected with hepatitis, and other wards had no residents with this infectious disease. I realized that such outbreaks were very contagious.

As a hospital surveyor, I knew perfect sanitary practice was very difficult to achieve. The kitchen supplied food to all the wards equally so it was evident the food was not the source of the hepatitis outbreak.

I noticed the personal sanitation of the mentally deficient children was poor despite the nursing staff's every effort. This was equally true of infected wards and uninfected wards. I concluded a child infected with the virus had been admitted to each ward that subsequently experienced an outbreak of hepatitis. Poor personal sanitary practices and shared food spread the disease. I recommended the isolation of infected children to one ward and, if possible, an emphasis on improved sanitary practices.

I had been in practice as a medical doctor a little over a year when the chief of staff at a local hospital appointed me to the chair of the infection control committee. Infectious disease specialists were rare in those days. I was assigned because I had degrees in bacteriology and public health, and I had experience as a hospital inspector before receiving my medical degree.

I soon had an important, but unpleasant, job. The hospital had experienced an outbreak of Staphylococcus infections in several postoperative patients and in the nursery. An investigation revealed the same general practitioner attended all these patients. Tests demonstrated that, though he himself was not ill, the same Staphylococcus that had infected his patients had colonized him.[19] He had become an agent of Staphylococcus transmission. Several of his activities had to be avoided. Without hesitation, he agreed to stop doing surgery and delivering infants until he was proven to be free of the offending germ.

Ridding him of the Staph proved to be tougher than expected. He finally went to the infectious disease professor at the local university, and there he was ultimately cleared of the organism.

Doctors had no idea then, that Staph would eventually colonize many patients, as well as many medical personnel. Transfer of germs, such as Staph, eventually lead to the development of universal precautions protocols, which can include the use

19 An individual is said to be "colonized" when he or she carries the germ in a body organ or orifice, but demonstrate no evidence of infection. Though not ill, the carrier may contaminate others with the germ. The individual, so contaminated, could then become infected.

of gloves, gowns, masks where indicated, and hand washing between each and every patient and procedure. In the hospital, everybody—nurses, visitors, doctors who are making their rounds—are now required to observe universal precautions.

When entering the room of a patient who is isolated because he or she has a contagious illness, the glove, gown, and mask rule applies. This rule extends beyond acute hospitals. It is also enforced at skilled nursing facilities. A germicide dispenser is in place at the door of each hospital room. Its use is required for all people who enter or leave the room. Dr. Semmelweis was right again!

WHAT IS INFORMED CONSENT?

In the late 1950s and 1960s, the doctrine of informed consent became a part of medical parlance. One major case involved one of my professors at USC School of Medicine, though the incident occurred elsewhere and not at the university or any facility affiliated with it. My professor, a neurosurgeon, saw a young Hispanic male at his office for pain and weakness of the lower extremities. The man spoke no English, so most of the conversation had to take place via an interpreter.

After examining the patient, the doctor decided it was necessary to rule out spinal cord involvement. He recommended a myelogram. This was in a time before noninvasive procedures such as CT scans or MRI were available. A myelogram consisted of the injection of a radiation opaque dye into the spinal column and taking X-rays of the back. The procedure was not without some discomfort and risk.

The patient is said to have asked if the test would be painful. My professor allegedly assured the patient that the only discomfort would be from lying on a cold, hard X-ray table and a small needle stick in the back.

The patient agreed to the procedure. Shortly after the procedure was completed, the patient complained he couldn't move his lower extremities.

In the malpractice suit that followed, several competent neurosurgeons testified that my professor and radiologist did nothing wrong. The symptoms described by the patient suggested he might have had a reaction to the contrast media that was injected. This is a rare, but possible, risk of the procedure. The episode could even represent an hysterical reaction manifested as paralysis. There also was the possibility that the underlying condition, the lumbar spinal problem, had caused the paralysis.

Although the neurosurgeon was not found guilty of any wrongdoing, the court decided the doctors and facility where the test was performed had failed to obtain the patient's informed consent to do the procedure. They did not tell the patient of the rare possibility of a reaction to the contrast media that could result in paralysis or even death. The requirement to inform the patient of every possible risk became known as the doctrine of informed consent, a principle that is true to this day.

MY FIRST EXPERIENCE WITH INFORMED CONSENT

Shortly after the case was described in the medical literature, one of my patients developed similar back and lower extremity pains, such as was described in my professor's case. I sent her to the hospital to have a myelogram done. About noon, I received a call from the radiologist. She was refusing the procedure. I rushed over to the hospital to ask her why she had refused the myelogram. She told me the radiologist told her of all the unlikely things that could happen to her so he could obtain her informed consent, as the courts had ruled. I explained all of the terrible things that the radiologist described really could happen, but, in fact, they happened very rarely. In spite of my explanation, she insisted on leaving the hospital without having the test.

A couple weeks later, she was back at my office. The pain medicines were not helping much. She stated she was a total invalid and would rather die than live in such misery. I again told her that spinal nerve roots were probably being pinched in her back and, if we could locate the spot with the aid of the myelogram, it could most likely be fixed.

I showed her the area where she was hurting in Frank Netter's book of medical illustrations as well as on a plastic model of the spine.[20] She finally agreed to undergo the procedure. The myelogram was performed without any problem. As suspected, she had a pinched nerve in her back. I then referred her to a neurosurgeon who successfully operated on her. The pain subsided. She went on to live comfortably and died years later of heart disease.

WHAT HAS HAPPENED TO INFORMED CONSENT?

The doctrine of informed consent still exists today, almost fifty years since the courts delineated it, but time constraints limit the amount of detail that the doctrine suggests. Detailed information often frightens patients, even though the likelihood of an untoward reaction might be rare. Written consents, which many patients sign, usually go unread.

The printed consent that patients always sign when they are admitted to the hospital is several pages long. I have never seen anyone read it. Verbal information may only address the most frequent adverse reactions and outcomes. When discussing a medicine or procedure with a patient, I describe the most likely reactions.

As I write this, I am reminded of a drug reaction that resulted in the death of one of my patients. I had

20 Frank H. Netter, *Nervous System* (1957), 49, 50, 113.

done a preoperative examination of this patient only six weeks earlier and found him in good health. He was on no medication. The operation, a corneal transplant, was successful. The ophthalmologist put the patient on a herpes-suppressing medication to prevent a virus infection from damaging the transplanted cornea.

Five weeks after surgery, he suddenly couldn't walk. Although he had been a healthy eighty-nine-year-old man, I was concerned he was having a stroke. I had him taken to the hospital. There, he was found to be in severe kidney failure, liver failure, and chemical imbalance.

The medicine the eye doctor had prescribed for him was commonly used in the medical community. None of the specialists I had called had ever heard of this medicine causing any significant side effects. But, when we looked up the adverse reactions of this medicine in the package insert, kidney failure was mentioned as a rare adverse reaction.

Despite every effort by the intensive care team, my patient died. His death was due to a commonly used, relatively innocuous drug. Even if an adverse reaction is rare, it's 100 percent for the person to whom it happens.

THE TUSKEGEE SYPHILIS STUDY

The classic study the United States Public Health Service performed on black males without proper informed consent was the Tuskegee Syphilis Study. In 1997, President Clinton formally apologized on behalf of the federal government to the African American population for this unjust treatment of those black males involved in the study. Informed consent wasn't the practice in those days. When penicillin became available and proved to be vastly superior to the older medications previously in use for treating syphilis, it was deliberately not utilized for the Tuskegee group in order to study the long-term effects of the untreated disease.

Not only is informed consent necessary for procedures and surgery, it's also important when prescribing medication. I don't want to frighten patients or put ideas into their heads. The power of suggestion is very convincing. That's why placebos work on some people. But a patient should know the downside of what he or she is putting into his or her system. Too often, the patient isn't told.

ANTIBIOTICS, THE WONDER DRUGS. I WONDER IF I NEED ONE?

The most famous story about antibiotics is the discovery of penicillin, which was found growing as a contaminant in a discarded Petri dish.[21] It was noticed that mold had overgrown in one of the dishes. This mold, later identified as the fungus Penicillium notatum, seemed to be inhibiting the growth of the bacteria that had been previously growing in the dish. The bacteria-inhibiting substance that the fungus was producing came to be known as penicillin.

During World War II, penicillin saved many lives, including that of my uncle. My uncle had double pneumonia (pneumonia affecting both lungs), a disease that frequently resulted in death in those days. A petition to the armed forces was required to release enough penicillin to save my uncle's life, or so his doctor told us.

The doctor's nurse had to make trips to my uncle's apartment every four hours to administer the injection, so the busy doctor seized the opportunity to teach me, the "future scientist," how to give penicillin injections. I

21 A Petri dish is a clear, covered dish that is three inches in diameter. It is filled with agar gelatin and used to grow bacteria for identification.

must admit I became dizzy and nauseated and couldn't perform that duty.

ANOTHER PENICILLIN "SHOT"

During World War II, I enlisted in the navy right out of high school, I'd been in the navy for less than a year when I developed a fungus infection all over my body and landed in the sick bay contagious disease ward. The sailor in the bed across from me had an abscessed ear.

Every day, the nurse would smear colored dyes and ointments on my entire body. She would then pour what she identified as sulfa powder into my ward mate's infected ear. When he didn't get better, she said he was going to get the new wonder drug named penicillin.

When it first became available, penicillin was an injection dissolved in beeswax. Every six hours, he was given a shot of penicillin deep into his buttock. It must have been very painful because he'd clutch the bed rail and howl every time he got the shot. He reminded the nurse that his abscess was in his "ear," not his "rear."

In those days, most injections were given in the upper arm. When we first came to active duty, we were given several immunizations (tetanus, typhoid, and so forth) in the arms. A penicillin shot was four times the volume of medicine contained in an immunization shot, and it had to be injected into a muscle big enough to handle the larger volume of medicine. So the buttocks muscle was used. The antibiotic era had begun!

THE CONSEQUENCES OF OVERUSING ANTIBIOTICES

By the time I became a doctor, antibiotics were already on the market. As time passed, many different antibiotics became available, and patients began to expect them for every infection. But an unexpected problem was brewing. Some bacteria, which antibiotics had easily controlled in the past, were becoming resistant. The pharmaceutical industry rose to the challenge by developing new antibiotics, but resistant strains of bacteria kept emerging. It seemed that bugs were smarter than we were.

The Centers for Disease Control and Prevention (CDC) warned us about this problem. They said the germs were becoming resistant because of the overuse of antibiotics. Several practices had to be avoided in order to minimize the emergence of resistant bacterial strains. Obviously, doctors should avoid prescribing antibiotics for illnesses that do not respond to antibiotics. This includes infections caused by fungi and viruses. Where there is infection by bacterial agents, cultures should be done in an effort to identify the infecting organism and decide which antibiotic would be the most effective.

Over the years, I have observed other practices that provide the patient with little or no benefit. When I started my practice, injectable penicillin was still being widely used. It was not uncommon for a patient to demand a shot of penicillin when oral medication, given over a period of days, could be just as effective or more so. Injections have no advantage over oral medicines unless:

- The patient is vomiting.
- The patient can't take anything by mouth.
- The patient is extremely ill.
- The antibiotic the patient needs doesn't come in an oral form.

Antibiotics are sometimes used to prevent infection from a possible exposure to infectious bacteria. There are some legitimate reasons for this. Some dental procedures risk contaminating the bloodstream with the patient's own bacteria. Cardiologists require dentists to use antibiotics if heart valve pathology is present. Contamination of the bloodstream could risk the infection of the heart. Orthopedic surgeons often advise the same precautions where infection-vulnerable hardware placed is in the body for joint reconstruction (an artificial hip). Other specific situations also require antibiotics. If prophylactic antibiotics are appropriate, the treating physician will so advise.

ALLERGY TO ANTIBIOTICS

Since the introduction of penicillin, millions of people have become allergic to it. The allergic reaction can be as minor as itching or light rash or as serious as anaphylaxis and death. You must tell your nurse or doctor if you are allergic to penicillin, or anything else you believe you are allergic to. To make things even more complicated, other substances with molecular relationship to penicillin, such as the cephalosporin family of antibiotics, may occasionally have cross-sensitive reactions with penicillin.

Before penicillin came on the scene, sulfa drugs were widely used to fight infections. New sulfa drugs have replaced the old preparations. They seem to be less allergenic, but millions of people, myself included, are still allergic to sulfa drugs. Many antibiotics are now available. Newer ones keep coming into the marketplace as the germs become resistant to the older ones.

Allergy is not the only hazard that entitles the antibiotics to be put into the all-medicines-are-poison family. As with all other medicines, antibiotics can cause numerous adverse reactions. Infections can cause serious illness, so there is usually less problem in weighing the benefit to be derived from taking an antibiotic against the risks that are involved, but the risks are there.

DO PLACEBOS HAVE A PLACE IN MEDICINE?

Every mother has the experience where her two-year-old takes a little fall and comes crying bitter tears. Mother sees there is no problem and says, "I'll kiss it and make it all better." After a kiss and a hug, the crying stops. That kiss is a placebo. The child believes Mother's kiss can make it better, so the child feels better after the (nonmedical) kiss.

On occasion, an elderly man will come to a doctor's office with some vague complaint and wants a prescription. An examination reveals no problem. The patient is well beyond the kissing cure. Some doctors will recommend an innocuous syrupy medicine (a placebo), and the patient goes home happy. Other doctors will say, "There's nothing wrong with you. Go home and get a good night's sleep." And maybe that doctor will lose a patient.

The dictionary definition describes a placebo as "a preparation that is pharmacologically inert but that may have a medical effect based solely on the power of suggestion." When I was young, many pharmacists were still preparing medications on an individual basis, following the doctor's written instructions (prescription). This was usually a liquid preparation or powder placed in capsules or folded papers. If a doctor wanted the patient to receive a placebo, it was relatively easy to disguise colored water, starch, or powdered sugar as an active medicine.

I could never bring myself to prescribe placebos. They have a place in medical research, but, in practice, I long ago decided that symptoms I believed to have no organic basis had to be dealt with honestly and up front. However, I do think that placebos work.

THE ART OF PRESCRIBING PLACEBOS

When I was in training at Los Angeles County General Hospital, I was aware the pharmacy prepared the syrup mixture of belladonna and phenobarbital in two colors, red and green. The outpatient department designated them as OPD 139 rubra (red) and OPD 139 verde (green). When rubra stopped working, we could prescribe verde. Without changing the medicine at all, simply by changing the color, we were successful in getting further usefulness and patient satisfaction out of the very same medicine.

OPD 139 was not a placebo. It contained active medicinal ingredients, but prescribing it in another color caused the patient to believe he or she was getting a different medicine, thus invoking the placebo effect. The placebo effect did seem to work, and the doctor avoided the risk of the side effects from a different medicine. (Remember that all medicines have side effects.)

A more important use of placebos is when evaluating the effectiveness of a new medicine or treatment procedure. The study population is divided into groups of similarly ill patients. One group is given the placebo; the other group is subjected to the treatment being tested. Neither the doctors nor the patients know which group is receiving treatment and which is getting the placebo.

IS THERE REALLY A PLACEBO AFFECT? IF YES, WHAT IS IT?

My colleague, Dr. Wallace Sampson, an oncologist and now retired professor of medicine at Stanford University, is still very active as a champion of reliable health information. He has a different viewpoint regarding placebos. He says there probably is no placebo effect. Every physician knows symptoms of illnesses wax and wane. Dr. Sampson points out that, when symptoms exacerbate, the patient is usually willing to take a medicine in order to obtain relief. When the patient feels better, he or she will often stop the medicine. If the medicine is a placebo, the patient may feel better because of the natural remission of the symptoms, not as a result of the placebo effect at all.

In all due respect, I cannot entirely agree with this view, although I believe it is one valid explanation of the placebo effect. I believe there are times when placebos actually alleviate the symptoms. The power of the mind is illustrated by the following excerpt from an article by Jay Dixit:

> "On the windowsill of his Columbia University office, psychiatrist B. Timothy Walsh has a little golden bottle labeled 'Placebo.' The container is filled with sugar pills -- breath mints, to be exact -- and purports to treat everything from 'bad hair' to 'can't take a joke' to 'no rhythm' to 'the blahs.' About 50 conditions are listed with a box next to each. The label directs patients: 'Select and check box. Take 2 mints. Bingo... all better.'
>
> Walsh's 'cure' is reminiscent of the snake oil, tonics and magical elixirs that used to be popular in this country -- the kind of carnival quackery that no one falls for anymore. Right? Well, not quite. According to a recent report by Seattle psychiatrist Arif

> Kahn, who conducted analysis of the placebo effect in 96 clinical trials submitted to the FDA between 1979 and 1996, sugar pills were often as effective as antidepressants."

Dixit writes that evidence indicates "a placebo study might show equal improvement to a medication group at first. But, if a placebo study were done over a period of several years, the placebo group would almost certainly fall behind." I agree with Dixit's article and B. Timothy Walsh's and Dr. Arif Kahn's report. In the long run, the real medicines will win out.

ARE PLACEBOS HARMLESS?

Placebos are harmless (if anything is), but, if the patient's illness is worthy of treatment with a real medication, the use of a placebo may actually be detrimental to his or her well-being.

The use of a placebo by a physician at a hospital where I am on staff became an issue recently. As chairman of the Biomedical Ethics Committee, I called a meeting to discuss this matter. The hospital's pharmacist declined to fill a physician's request to provide the placebo for use in his patient. The patient had asked for a medicine that the doctor decided she shouldn't have.

The basis for denial of the request was twofold. First, the pharmacist believed the use of placebos violated the doctrine of informed consent. The doctrine of informed consent requires a patient be fully and honestly informed about the treatment, its benefits, and adverse reactions. Second, no placebos were available at the hospital pharmacy, nor were any available to order.

During the discussion of the issues, I pointed out that placebo use was a traditional practice of medicine. Many doctors felt it had a legitimate role. In my opinion, although it would require a change of the hospital's admission documents, the possible use of placebos by the physicians who attended to patients at the hospital should be written into the informed consent, which all patients signed when they were admitted. The purpose of doing this is not to hide that information in a document that everybody signs but nobody reads. It becomes part of the informed consent and qualifies as the patient's legitimate agreement to a treatment process. But the hospital attorney advised against that. Needless to say, his opinion prevailed.

If placebos work (and I personally believe they do), then the patient must not be aware that he or she is receiving a placebo. Placebos work because the patient believes he or she is taking a real medicine.

DOSAGE COUNTS: START LOW AND GO SLOW

Many articles and even books have been written proclaiming that doctors tend to prescribe too many medicines (polypharmacy). Medicines are sometimes prescribed at too high a dose. My professor of pharmacology warned us to "start low and go slow" when prescribing. But there are times when this admonition doesn't apply. The best example of that involves the prescribing of antibiotics. Doctors are aware that, when prescribing antibiotics, enough must be given to prevent the survival of the resistant bacteria and emergence of a resistant strain. In the case of tuberculosis, it has been found necessary to use several antibiotics concurrently. At the time this is written, no one antibiotic will eliminate the tubercle bacillus from the human body. It may require four!

TOO LITTLE, TOO MUCH, OR JUST RIGHT

Just as too little of a medicine may be ineffective or even dangerous; too much can also be dangerous. Unnecessarily excessive dosage is not only wasteful, but it increases the incidence and intensity of adverse reactions. Over the years during which I have been in practice, I have seen prescription medicines cause my patients unacceptable side effects, even when I was careful to prescribe the lowest therapeutic dose. When necessary, I recommended reducing the dosage by splitting the pill or opening the capsule and dividing the contents into two doses.

My patients complained about intolerable side effects that a newly released antidepressant caused, even though I had prescribed the lowest dose tablet. I brought this problem to the attention of the local representative of the pharmaceutical company. I was soon pleased to see a new, lower dosage form arrive on the market. I have no doubt that many physicians were reporting similar experiences that demonstrated the need for the lower dosage.

Years ago, I discovered I could prescribe diuretics for hypertension at lower dosages than what were available at the time and still get good results. My patients who followed this advice often experienced fewer side effects caused by low potassium and sodium.

While driving to a medical meeting with one of my cardiology consultants, he commented that I was prescribing the diuretic medicines at a lower dosage than the accepted practice of the time. I responded that they seemed to be working well at the lower dosage. I predicted the pharmaceutical manufacturers would discover this fact and eventually make lower-dosage pills. Meanwhile, I continued to have my patients split them. In time, lower doses became the standard.

Some physicians were very concerned about the excessive dosage levels that the pharmaceutical industry recommended for their medications. Several articles regarding this issue have appeared in the medical literature. At least two books have been written about the subject. I recently read a book entitled *Overdose* that addressed the issue.[22] I have also noticed that several drugs have become available in new lower dosage forms, usually with no decrease in price.

---

22 Jay Cohen, MD, *Overdose* (Penguin Putnam, Inc.).

IMMUNIZATIONS

The story of immunization has many chapters impacted by the risk versus benefit issues. In the nearly sixty years during which I have been involved in the health and medical care fields, there have been amazing advances. But there have also been some bumps in the road. When I was in training at Los Angeles County General Hospital, I remember a room full of idle respirator tanks (iron lungs). They had been primarily designed for paralyzed poliomyelitis patients who could no longer breathe on their own. The Salk and Sabin vaccines changed that, but not without some glitches along the way.

Prior to the Salk and Sabin vaccines, paralytic poliomyelitis was also known as infantile paralysis. It attacked so many small children and infants that it kept those respirator tanks busy. My uncle had a withered lower limb from a childhood bout with polio and limped the rest of his life. President Roosevelt was confined to a wheelchair and used braces and crutches by what was said to be the result of polio. As president, he promoted the March of Dimes, the proceeds of which helped fund polio research.

When Jonas Salk perfected his polio vaccine, the whole country lined up for polio shots. As a young doctor, I volunteered to supervise free polio vaccine injection clinics that were held at banks, schools, and hospitals in the San Fernando Valley, where I lived and worked.

In the early days of the campaign, there was a problem with some of the vaccine. A pharmaceutical company unintentionally released a batch of Salk polio vaccine that still had some live virus in it. The Salk vaccine was designed as a killed virus injection that was not supposed to contain any live virus. A number of the vaccine's recipients developed polio. This incident almost scuttled the pharmaceutical manufacturer as well as the vaccination campaign. But the problem was solved. Live Salk virus was never again allowed to slip through the manufacturing process.

By the time I was supervising the San Fernando Valley clinics in my area, everything went smoothly. Salk vaccine ushered the iron lung and braces into medical history. However, there is a sequence and, unfortunately, another glitch in the polio vaccine story.

While Dr. Salk was perfecting the polio vaccine injection, Dr. Albert Sabin was working on a live oral polio vaccine. Many people do not like shots but would not mind swallowing an oral vaccine. The oral vaccine was live poliovirus that had been modified (attenuated) so it no longer caused the disease, but it resembled the wild disease-causing virus enough to fool the human body into making protective antibodies against polio. The oral polio vaccine quickly replaced the Salk vaccine as the preferred way of immunizing against poliomyelitis infection.

Then disaster loomed again. It was found that children immunized with the live, attenuated Sabin virus could spread poliovirus that had reverted into a virulent form. This was a very rare event. The children who received the Sabin vaccine didn't get polio, but some of the grandparents, who had never been immunized (and had no immunity to poliovirus), did contract polio after they had spent time with their Sabin vaccine-immunized grandchildren who were spreading live, contagious polio virus.

When public health authorities discovered this phenomenon, the obvious solution was to return to immunization with Salk's killed virus vaccine. The current practice is to immunize with Salk vaccine first and then either stay with Salk or go to Sabin later after the child has developed some immunity. But nobody can predict if that pattern will be changed again. In medicine, for every benefit, there's always a risk. Some risks defy prediction.

MORE VACCINATION PROBLEMS

Some years ago, a British physician noted some of the infants immunized with the pertussis (whooping cough) vaccine had a prolonged shrieking/crying spell after the injection of the vaccine. It was postulated (but not proved) that the vaccine could induce brain damage in some infants. This report was publicized in England. It so frightened mothers of infants that many of them refused to have their children immunized. The increased pool of children susceptible to whooping cough resulted in an epidemic that caused far more harm than the bad outcomes that the immunization campaign might have caused.

In my own practice, an occasional child did not tolerate the pertussis vaccine and exhibited the "shrieking" symptom. I decided the better part of wisdom was to discontinue the immunization with the vaccine we had available at that time. The pharmaceutical industry discovered the cellular component of the vaccine was causing the problem. They developed an acellular vaccine, which was just as effective, but didn't cause the problem.

A DESPERATE NEED FOR A NEW VACCINE

During World War I, thousands of cases of tetanus were among the casualties because of contamination of their wounds by Clostridium tetani, a normal resident in the environment and especially in some fertilizers. By the time World War II started, all military personnel were required to be immunized with tetanus vaccine. Only seven cases were reported during the entire war. The vaccine is so effective that one wonders if those seven people actually received the vaccine. To maintain its protective benefits, tetanus vaccine should be boosted every ten years if the patient has not had a susceptible wound. A person who sustains a deep, ragged, or dirty wound susceptible to tetanus should get a booster shot if he or she has not had one within five years.

I became aware that a wound might not always be a necessary prerequisite of a tetanus infection. One of my elderly patients developed symptoms suggestive of tetanus, but had experienced no significant wound. He had been gardening a few days earlier and became covered with manure fertilizer dust. Manure is known to have a high content of the tetanus organism. He had not had a tetanus vaccine since he was in the service almost fifty years earlier.

I suspected it might be tetanus, so I sent him to the USC infectious disease service at Los Angeles County General Hospital. They did diagnose tetanus and treated him with tetanus antitoxin. He recovered. He was very lucky, but, if he had received a tetanus immunization every ten years, he wouldn't have needed that luck.

Tetanus is a deadly disease, but people have been known to be allergic to the tetanus antitoxin that saved my patient's life. For those people, the risk of taking the antitoxin outweighed the risk of getting tetanus. This represents another example of how medicines can be poison in unanticipated ways.

ETHICAL ISSUES IN MEDICINE

ADVERTISING: THE HIGH COST OF PROMOTION

When I was an undergraduate in college, a classmate and I were seriously planning to go into the field of developing specific vaccines for the immunization of patients whose own immune system was having difficulty dealing with infection. I was a bacteriology major; my friend was a chemistry major. It was just after the end of World War II. Only a few antibiotics were on the market. Persistent bacterial and viral infections sometimes yielded to specific immune serum therapy, so the field seemed to be wide open for two young, enthusiastic minds. Our plan was to produce immune-specific serums to help control infections in patients whose own immunity was failing to do the job.

We didn't count on the rapidity at which new antibiotics were arriving on the market. Resistance of microorganisms to antibiotics was still rare at that time, so every new antibiotic seemed to be a knockout blow for the infectious germs. We decided the demand for specific vaccines was not going to be as large as we first expected so I went on to a career in public health and then the private practice of family medicine. My classmate went on to earn a PhD in chemistry and then to a successful career in research.

THE ETHICAL DRUG COMPANIES

In the 1940s and 1950s, the pharmaceutical producers were known as the ethical drug companies. They earned this appellation because their research efforts were done ethically and conclusions were based strictly upon the evidence-based, double-blind research. In those days, the pharmaceutical industry advertised their prescription products only to the health care industry, not the general public.

I haven't heard the expression "ethical drug company" used in years. In my opinion, a number of things have happened since the industry was thought of as ethical. I do understand the need for profits. The pharmaceutical industry takes significant financial risks to develop valuable new medicines. Many of these products fail to ever achieve the FDA requirements that allow them to reach the market. Marketing is also an expensive and complicated process with no assurance of success. But some of the industry's profit-motivated tactics have gone beyond what I regard as ethical.

A PROGRAM THAT BACKFIRED

The 1992 Prescription Drug User Fee Act authorized the FDA to collect fees from companies that produced drugs and biologicals for human use. These fees were intended to make it possible for the FDA to expedite drug reviews by hiring more personnel, thus permitting earlier approval.

Prior to this new law, the government paid for the entire cost of product overview by the FDA. The new fee program seemed like a good idea, but, in my opinion, it has backfired. It appears to me that the FDA has allowed the pharmaceutical industry to push it into releasing some drugs before they are fully studied. The FDA has had to withdraw an increasing number of medicines from the market after they had been released. The FDA also admits they have not been able to adequately respond to reports of adverse events.

The *Wall Street Journal* had some editorials regarding FDA policies with which they disagreed. One, "FDA to Patients: Drop Dead," argues that critically ill patients with diseases such as AIDS will die if possibly life-saving drugs are required to go through the full FDA study protocol before being marketed.[23] This is probably true, but, without the full study protocol, severe and even

23 "FDA to Patients: Drop Dead," *Wall Street Journal*, 24 September 2002.

deadly unexpected effects may not be discovered. A drug, which might finally be determined to be relatively ineffective, could kill more people than it saved.

The discovery of unexpected and dangerous effects of new drugs after they have been approved for marketing to the public has always been a problem, even before fast tracking. Since Congress has encouraged the more rapid approval of new medicines by the FDA, a greater number of drugs have had to be taken off the marketplace because of the identification of serious side effects.

WHEN MARKETING AND MEDICINE COLLIDE

Another practice where ethics have been questioned is direct marketing to the consumer. The obvious intent is to create a demand for a particular drug by name. This encourages patients to request medicines that may not be best suited for their needs. Busy, well-meaning physicians may acquiesce to a patient's request for a particular medication, even though it may not be the one the physician would have preferred to prescribe. On the other hand, many doctors welcome drug advertising to the public in the belief that it educates the public and makes their prescribing decisions easier. However, a vigorous advertising campaign will likely also increase the cost of the medicine.

The pharmaceutical manufacturers concurrently employ thousands of representatives whose job is to convince the doctors that their products are the best. Price is never mentioned unless their product is less expensive than the competitor's. In addition to advertising to the consumer, multiple-page advertisements also appear in numerous professional journals in an effort to reinforce the impression that theirs is the best available drug in that specific class.

FOCUS GROUP DISCUSSIONS

Another pharmaceutical industry practice of questionable ethics is the funding of focus group discussions where physicians are invited to a dinner meeting, usually at a local hotel or restaurant, to listen to and participate in a presentation that focuses on the virtues of one of the products sold by the company. It's not uncommon to discuss off-label uses at these meetings. Physicians are permitted to prescribe for off-label uses, but the FDA does not permit the pharmaceutical industry to promote off-label use.

The physicians are enticed to the meeting by the promise of a medical supply item or book gift with the value of about $100. This gift meets the maximum value permitted by AMA guidelines and is not considered being an enticement to prescribe.[24] However, this issue is not the worrisome one. The FDA requires that any discussion of a prescription medicine by a drug company representative must not deviate from the facts described in the product brochure.

Someone who isn't an employee of the manufacturer often moderates the focus groups. The moderator makes a presentation to start the discussion and then urges every participant to make comments regarding his or her experience with the product and his or her impression of it. This often leads to comments about off-label uses and tends to emphasize positive results and diminish negative effects. I suspect a focused discussion at a medical conference moderated by an unbiased university professor would have a somewhat different thrust. It's now required that, prior to giving the presentation, speakers at accredited medical education meetings must state their affiliations and any financial arrangements they may have with the pharmaceutical industry.

The dinner meetings are still continuing, but some of the pharmaceutical companies, in an effort to add legitimacy to their meetings, are no longer offering a monetary gift for attending. Some of the meetings offer continuing medical education credit. Physicians are

24 The AMA may soon lower the allowable stipend to $50.

required to document a minimum number of continuing medical education hours each three years. These meetings are an easy way to obtain them, but it probably isn't the best way.

WHY PRESCRIPTION DRUGS COST SO MUCH?

Many of the prescription drugs on the market today were developed with substantial financial support and expertise from federal government agencies in the Department of Health and Human Services. Medicines have been developed in the research laboratories of other countries, including England, France, Germany, Switzerland, and Italy. Until recent years, most medicines developed in the United States were researched and studied prior to release at the laboratories of the universities and major drug companies.

It has been widely publicized that it is extremely expensive to develop a new medicine because of the cost of the research and the fact that many new products never reach the market and are a complete loss financially. While this is true, it's not the sole reason prescription medicines are so expensive in the United States.

The pharmaceutical manufacturing industry wants the public to believe that most of the cost of producing a new drug is research and manufacturing. However, marketing to the prescribing doctors, advertising to the public, large profit margins, and the industry's practice of producing copycat drugs all contribute heavily to the price of medicines. Research and development costs pale in comparison, though the pharmaceutical industry denies it.

Marketing alone has been an increasing burden on the cost of prescription medication in recent years. There are several aspects to marketing. The initial marketing of a prescription medication is to the physicians who will be prescribing the product. Pharmaceutical firms employ thousands of representatives who visit the doctors at their offices, hospitals, and medical meetings. They are supposed to detail the benefits and risks of the drug they represent, but, too often, they dwell on the benefits and minimize the risks.

During these visits, samples of the medications are left, and the doctor is usually given various small gifts, such as pens, pads, and other trinkets. Each of which is emblazoned with the drug name and manufacturer's logo. In past years, larger gifts such as trips to meetings at resort hotels, sports events, and retreats have been given to doctors and their families. Those days remind me of the Washington lobbyists who influenced the United States Congress to pass laws favorable to the pharmaceutical industry. The AMA, in an effort to defend the ethical and professional standing of physicians, discourages accepting gifts exceeding a value of $100. The AMA has published guidelines for what is acceptable, such as educational meetings funded by the pharmaceutical industry. However, every speaker must acknowledge any relationship with or remuneration by that industry.

Another method is the focused discussion session. A group of practicing physicians is invited to a dinner meeting or conference call where a speaker discusses a single product. A round table discussion follows. During which, the physicians share anecdotes and experiences about the medicine being discussed. Every doctor is encouraged to comment. Some of the things said at these sessions would not meet the approval of the FDA if they were published in an advertisement. The hook used to persuade the physicians to participate in these sessions is an honorarium in the form of a medical book or piece of office equipment valued at about $100. In the face of the ethical issues described above, the $100 award is also disappearing, although I was recently offered a $250 honorarium for participating in a two- to three-hour conference at a nearby hotel.

Concurrent with direct-to-physician marketing are advertisements in medical journals and other periodicals distributed to physicians and hospitals. These are rarely single-page ads. Some are actually four to eight pages in length and in a glossy, multicolored display. They are usually accompanied by a full, detailed description, which the FDA requires, in tiny, almost unreadable, type at the end of the advertisement. Lately, I have been receiving numerous popular magazines at my office. All of which are replete with medicine advertisements. They are obviously intended to be displayed in my waiting room and possibly read by me. I did not ask for these magazines nor do I pay for them. I can only assume that it's either an attempt to promote magazine subscriptions or the pharmaceutical industry is trying to promote its products. Maybe it's both.

In recent years, the pharmaceutical companies have been advertising prescription drugs directly to the public on radio, television, and lay print media, urging patients to ask their doctor to prescribe the product being promoted. This practice is primarily a profit-building process for the pharmaceutical industry, which adds to the cost of medicines and adds little or no benefit for the patient.

Another activity that increases the cost of medicines to the patient is the number of intermediaries between the manufacturer and patient. In the past, only two levels were between the patient and manufacturerer, the wholesaler and the retailer. Each level that deals with getting a medicine to the patient is entitled to a profit.

The manufacturer usually depends on a wholesaler to distribute its product to the retailer, a retail pharmacy, hospital pharmacy, or clinic. The advent of health maintenance organizations (HMOs) resulted in the development of prescription benefit management programs (PBMs). The duty of a prescription benefit manager is to decide which medicines will be listed in the HMO's formulary (list of which medicines that would be paid for).

Usually, there is at least one medication from each class of drugs. Different medications in the same class are often very similar in action, and the patient is usually well-served by most of them. Older medications, where the patent has expired, are frequently offered only as their generic equivalent. Each PBM publishes a unique formulary of medications that are made available to the patients who have selected or been assigned to their program by the HMO or insurance company.

Some of the large purchasers of medication will not only insist on the lowest price from the manufacturer, but will negotiate with several manufacturers of medications of the same class of drugs. The least expensive medicine in the class often becomes the drug of choice. The patient on the plan will thus be able to obtain formulary drugs at a lower cost than medications not listed in the formulary.

The problems surface when a patient or physician decides not to use the drug that has been selected for the formulary. If a doctor has a legitimate reason for selecting a different, though similar, drug, there is an appeal system. It sometimes works, but it takes extra time and paperwork.

Over one hundred million American patients have prescription benefit cards, allowing them to obtain prescription medicines at a reduced price, but the medicine must be on the formulary list. The federal government recently discovered the PBMs are making secret deals for a fee, in exchange for positioning that company's brand of medication on the PBM's formulary as the drug of choice. In reality, that medicine may have no particular advantage over the other medications in its class, but it may actually cost the patient more.

The presence as the drug of choice on the formulary implies to both the patient and the doctor that the medicine is better than, just as good as, or less expensive than those not listed. For this reason, doctors are usually willing to prescribe the formulary-preferred drug for the patient, but not always. If the doctor chooses to prescribe a medicine that is not on the formulary, the insurance carrier will eventually inform the patient that the prescribed drug is not on the formulary and ask, but cannot require, the prescription be changed. If the doctor insists on continuing with the non-formulary medicine, then the patient may be required to pay more for it.

Occasionally, an insurance company will pay for a medication that is not on its formulary if the doctor is willing to write a convincing letter explaining why the patient must have the non-formulary medication. But because it's difficult for most doctors to find the time to write the letter or fill out the form, it is seldom done. So the patient pays more for his or her medicine, even though he or she has a prescription plan.

However, the person who really gets stuck is the patient without a paid prescription plan. All this bickering over price results in cost-shifting (the practice of charging people without insurance more to offset the discounts they give to the insurance program). The manufacturer still wants to earn higher profits than competitive bidding permits, so the cost of the medication on the open market rises to fill the gap.

The Part D prescription benefit program that was added to Medicare and Medicaid in 2005 permitted private, for-profit, insurance companies to create formularies. Part D also required the pharmacies to collect a copayment fee that Medicaid patients previously did not have to pay. Medicaid patients include some of the poorest people in our society. Some cannot even afford to pay the nominal additional prescription fee.

The Part D program became active in January 2006. It's a disgrace that Congress did not allow the Medicare system to negotiate medicine prices. Every other health care insurance (unsurance) program does. Whatever pharmceutical savings most Part D participants gained, increasing medicine prices has already neutralized them.

In response to the fact that numerous doctors were having denials by Part D providers for medicines the doctors preferred, the *American Medical News* published an article telling doctors to keep trying because the Part D law allows five levels of appeal. My own negative experiences when I appealed to the Part D insurance carriers persuaded me to reply to the *American Medical News* article with a letter to the editor that I entitled, "Five Levels of No!" It was published.

THE PROBLEM OF COPYCAT DRUGS

The prescription formularies reveal another factor that inflates the cost of medicine, redundancy. When a pharmaceutical manufacturer comes up with a new, unique medication, it stands to make a tidy profit on it because there is no competition. If the new drug proves to be successful, other pharmaceutical company laboratories endeavor to produce chemical structures very much like the breakthrough drug, but modified slightly so they are entitled to a patent of their own. This knockoff will have essentially similar effects, but, because it is constituted of a slightly changed molecule, the FDA is willing to approve it. It is then marketed as a different, new drug.

These medicines are known as "congeners." Doctors often call them me-too drugs. I have no objection to these medications if they bring an advantage that was not available from the original substance. Improvement is always welcome, whether it be greater efficacy, fewer adverse reactions, or longer duration. But, if the congener is no more than an imitation, it is more likely to increase cost rather than reduce it. This is due to the necessity of competitive marketing programs as well as the research that permitted it to come to market.

Extended release forms of some multi-dosage medicines permit longer duration of activity and make it easier to take medicine. The patients may then be able to take their medicine less often and are less likely to forget a dose. That is not always desirable. Drug company advertising tries to convince the doctors and patients that it is. The therapeutic benefits last longer, but so do the adverse reactions.

Congeners are not to be confused with generic drugs. Generic drugs are never available until the original, exclusive patent for a new drug runs out. The generic products are chemically identical to the original molecule. They are usually less expensive than the brand-name drug because the producer didn't have the expense of the original research, development, and marketing. Subsequent modifications of a new drug molecule does require adherence to the FDA's research and development protocol, no matter how small a change there is in the molecular configuration, so they may be just as expensive as the original item and often are.[25]

---

25 An excellent discussion of many of the issues covered by this chapter, as well as other problems with PBMs that are not detailed here, is addressed by John Carroll's article, "When Success Sours: PBMs Under Scrutiny." It appeared in the September 2002 issue of *Managed Care*.

TREATMENT OPTIONS CHANGE FREQUENTLY

While there is no doubt that all medicines should be prescribed with serious consideration of the risks and benefits, this principle also applies to other treatment modalities.

HOW MEDICAL TREATMENT ADVANCES AFFECT PATIENT OUTCOMES

Both my father and cousin had rheumatic heart problems long before I became a doctor. My cousin's heart had been so severely damaged by rheumatic heart disease that he spent the rest of his life as an invalid. While I was still in medical school, the heart-lung machine was being perfected. One of the hospitals in Los Angeles was doing open-heart surgeries. My cousin's parents realized he needed this surgery in order to correct the damaged heart valve. The risks of the surgery were still very high in those days, so the family doctor suggested they delay surgery until the risks were reduced. My cousin died in his late thirties of his heart disease before the surgery was perfected. Some patients were surviving heart surgery then, but the risk was still high. Would he have been one of the survivors? We'll never know.

Fortunately, my father's disease was mild and did not cause serious symptoms until he was in his seventies. At which time, he had to have his defective heart valve replaced. The operation extended his life and reinstated his health. He lived to be ninety and died of something else.

Open-heart surgery was a relatively safe procedure by the time my father had his operation. The equipment had been perfected; the surgeons had already operated on thousands of cases. There were still risks, poor outcomes, and even deaths, but the risk ratio was much better. Today, most heart surgery is successful.

AMAZING NEW DIAGNOSTIC MODALITIES AND TREATMENTS

Treatment options continue to advance. Many surgical procedures are less invasive. Laparoscopic surgery uses miniature television camera probes and buttonhole-sized incisions for inserting the necessary cutting, clamping, and grasping instruments into the body. Inaccessible areas of the small bowel are now being visualized by swallowing a small capsule that contains a tiny television camera, light, battery, and transmitter that relays images to an external receiver.

The receiver records hundreds of images as the capsule traverses the small bowel.

The gamma knife accurately destroys brain tumors without harming normal brain tissue and surgically opening the skull. The gamma knife is a beam of radiation that is electronically focused on the tumor.

Numerous other treatment and diagnostic advances have been developed since I finished medical school. As with all medicines, all treatments, surgical and otherwise, must be evaluated on the basis of benefits versus risks.

CHELATION THERAPY

Years ago, it was my good fortune to meet the doctor who first conceived of chelation therapy. He was giving a talk at a diabetic fund-raiser. Although his subject was diabetes, he shared the story of how he stumbled onto chelation therapy. As he told it, he was working in the pharmacy of a university teaching hospital one night when a request came down from the pediatric treatment unit regarding a child who was in the hospital suffering from heavy metal poisoning. In those days, lead paint was commonly used in homes. They are now illegal for that use in this country because, in the past, many small children ingested the paint on the fixtures and furniture of their dwelling and developed lead poisoning.[26]

The resident physician on duty at hospital that night was asking for a treatment for the child's heavy metal intoxication (lead poisoning). In those days, our speaker told us, there was no treatment for lead poisoning.

After giving the request some thought, our speaker recalled that there was a commercial agent that captured heavy metals and bound them tightly (sequestered them) so that they were rendered inactive. He obtained some of this agent and filtered it through a Berkfeld filter in order to sterilize it.

A Berkfeld filter is capable of removing tiny particles, even those as small as bacteria. He then calculated the amount of lead in the child's body and sent up enough material for injection to remove the toxic lead. Voila! Sequestration treatment for heavy metals was born. Allegedly, the child recovered from the lead poisoning. This procedure is now known as chelation therapy.

That was many years ago before the FDA regulated such matters. I hasten to state that the FDA currently has strict regulations about how new treatments and

26 Lead in the paints used on children's toys is now illegal in the United States. Recently, many toys imported from China were found to be colored with lead paint. Millions had to be removed from toy store shelves.

medicines can be used. An experiment such as this would never be allowed today, nor should be.

ANOTHER ASPECT OF CHELATION

I relate the following report to bring out another aspect of chelation treatment. Some medical practitioners use chelation therapy as a method of reducing cholesterol levels, clogged heart arteries, and other angiosclerotic diseases. There has been no scientifically validated evidence that chelation therapy is of any use in the human body other than for removing toxic heavy metals such as lead or arsenic.

I am unaware that an FDA-supervised, double-blind, evidence-based human study has ever successfully been done that uses chelation therapy for anything other than heavy metal poisoning. Physicians offering chelation for other purposes than heavy metal poisoning are working outside of the standards of good medical practice.[27]

27 A position paper regarding chelation is available on the National Council Against Health Fraud Web site at www.ncahf.org. It clarifies the approved and unapproved use of chelation therapy.

DOING NOTHING

A most difficult thing to do in the practice of medicine is nothing. When I am convinced that my diagnosis is correct and doing nothing will be just as effective as resorting to a medication or treatment process, I allow the healing process of the body to proceed by itself. The hands-off policy of doing nothing becomes my treatment. The decision to do nothing is actually doing something, such as not prescribing an antibiotic for a viral infection. Most of my patients understand why I sometimes choose not to prescribe, cut, or otherwise treat. When I explain why, they usually go along with it.

Some doctors find doing nothing so difficult because, when patients come to a doctor, they expect to receive a treatment for their ailments. I have known doctors who give B12 injections just to fulfill the patient's need to have something done when nothing would do fine. B12 is a valuable medicine to use with a pernicious anemia patient, but it is generally of little or no value for most common illnesses. However, a shot may have a powerful placebo effect. A B12 injection is relatively safe, and the patient's need for medical treatment is satisfied.

DOING NOTHING CAN BE A VALUABLE AND SAFE TREATMENT

Providing no treatment isn't really doing nothing. It is reassurance there will be a favorable outcome without exposing the patient to the risks that may accompany a treatment modality. The patient is not really coming to the doctor for medicine or a shot; the patient is coming for consultation and advice. Appropriate medical advice that recommends waiting for the body to heal itself has been known medically as tincture of time. It is worth the fee, just as is the surgeon who correctly decides an operation isn't necessary.

I proudly recall a case where that actually happened. A teenage patient developed a painful mass in the back of her right knee. I referred her to an orthopedic surgeon, who was perplexed and concerned about the mass. This was in the era before MRIs and CT scans, which would have clearly diagnosed the problem. Worried about a possible tumor, he decided to operate and explore the area. She was put under a general anesthetic. As soon as she was fully anesthetized, the mass disappeared. After careful closed examination of the knee, the surgeon decided to forgo the surgery. He was convinced she had a severe and persistent muscle spasm that subsided under deep anesthesia. This diagnosis proved to be true. The parents were grateful that we chose not to treat. But perhaps we did. Anesthesia is a powerful muscle relaxant. Today, we would have the advantage of soft tissue imaging devices to assure us that there is no tumor. Powerful muscle relaxants are now available if needed.

LAYING ON OF HANDS

We have discussed the risks of medicines at length. What about the risks of other forms of intervention? In the healing arts, we refer to the value of the laying on of hands. This includes massage, manipulation, and application of various physical modalities, such as ultrasound, diathermy, heat, and cold. Unfortunately, these methods, which have their place and admittedly usually feel good, can also do harm. I have taken care of patients after they had manipulation that made their pain worse than it was before. One of my patients was suffering from torn tissues and cracked cartilage of the neck, apparently due to chiropractic manipulation. Heat and diathermy (a high-frequency current generator device) can be comforting and beneficial, but it can also cause burns and discomfort if not used carefully. Physical modalities of treatment have their place, but not where no other treatment will work just as well. As discussed earlier, placebos can also provide pain relief and comfort at least for a time.

LEARNING AN IMPORTANT LESSON

The practice of withholding treatment when none is indicated reminds me of an incident that occurred while I was still in training. A physician, a successful obstetrician in South America, came to the United States to practice. In order to get his license here, he had to take a further residency in an accredited American facility. We, the interns at that hospital, had the benefit of his extensive past experience.

One day, a woman came to our labor suite in active labor with her fetus in a breech position. The head was up, and the buttocks were facing the pelvic outlet. The issue was whether we should attempt to turn the fetus to a head-down position before performing the delivery. We called our South American colleague to consult. He assessed the situation and promptly announced, "We will perform the hands in the pockets procedure!" We took his advice. The patient delivered a healthy baby by means of a breech delivery.

OTHER TREATMENTS THAT SOMETIMES WORK BUT ARE ACTUALLY DOING NOTHING

Therapeutic touch, a procedure where a therapist waves his or her hands over the patient's reclining body, is actually touchless. This therapy and other touchless modalities, when subjected to scientific investigation, may be doing nothing, but they sometimes seem to work. The mind and the body are often able to heal themselves. There's also the reassurance factor operating with these modalities.

When I recommend no treatment, I always explain that it's sometimes sensible to allow the body to heal itself and why it could be the best and safest route to recovery. That's the reassurance factor and it should be regarded as a form of treatment.

When I don't prescribe a specific treatment, I also tell my patients to call me if they don't feel better in a reasonable period of time. If they do not achieve a complete return to health, I may elect to prescribe a medication or other treatment. But where no treatment is required, I do nothing.

CONFLICTS OF INTERESTS: HOW THEY AFFECT YOUR HEALTH

The United States Government Manual depicts the Department of Health and Human Services by means of an inverted tree branch schematic.[28] Several branches are responsible for the financing and oversight of many of the matters discussed in this book. Among those subunits are:

- The CDC studies disease trends and acts as an early warning system for epidemics.
- The National Institutes of Health (NIH) overviews and funds medical, complementary, and alternative medical research.
- The FDA determines that patients and their doctors have access to a broad spectrum of safe medicines.

There have been several news reports that many physicians and scientists employed by the NIH and FDA receive honoraria from the industries they are responsible for reviewing and regulating. This is for lecturing or co-authoring articles. I have no objection to an FDA doctor supplementing his income by working in an unrelated

28 *United States Government Manuel, 2003–2004* (Government Printing Office).

field. This will not influence his or her judgment as a scientist. However, if part of his income comes from the industry he or she is responsible for regulating, it might influence his or her decision-making.

I was troubled by a news report regarding FDA doctors who approved the drug Rezulin over the objections of at least one FDA physician. He noted that, prior to its approval, the drug had caused serious end-stage liver damage. This resulted in some patient deaths. I wrote a letter to the editor of the *New York Times*, the newspaper that broke the story. In my letter, I complained I feared for my patients who used a medicine not properly evaluated by the FDA.

Shortly thereafter, the FDA authorities decided to remove Rezulin from the market. In view of the known end-stage liver damage Rezulin could cause, it probably shouldn't have been on the market in the first place.

EMPLOYEES OF REGULATING AGENCIES SHOULDN'T ACCEPT PAY FROM THE INDUSTRY THEY ARE REGULATING

The NIH is responsible for regulating much of the health and medical research done in the United States. When the story in the *New York Times* broke, the director of the NIH admitted the NIH did not require that its employees reveal remunerations received from the industry it regulated. A blue-ribbon committee was investigating this.

I wrote a letter to the editor of the *New York Times*, pointing out that receiving money from the industry that an individual is responsible for regulating constitutes a conflict of interest. If NIH scientists received money from the industry they were supervising, the NIH should not only know it, but this information should also be available to the public. In my letter, I stated that such activity shouldn't be allowed. You either work for the government or an industry that is regulated by your government job, but not for both!

Subsequently, *Family Practice News* published an article stating that external and internal reviews led the NIH to recommend "deep changes in the agency's conflict of interest policies."[29] These recommendations proposed that all NIH employees be prohibited from receiving or holding stocks or stock options in biotechnology or pharmaceutical companies as compensation for research and consulting. The agency will also require employees to disclose their compensated activities with outside groups.

Apparently, the NIH has failed to achieve its goal. In 2006, at least two NIH doctors admitted to be accepting

29 Mary Ellen Schneider, "Director Proposes Tougher Ethics Rules for NIH Scientists," *Family Practice News* 14 no. 17 (September 2004).

funds from the pharmaceutical industry to the tune of hundreds of thousands of dollars. One NIH doctor admitted he gave more than a thousand NIH tissue samples[30] to the private industry without the knowledge or permission of the Institute.

There are reports that literally hundreds of FDA and NIH employees collect consulting fees (as much as $300,000 per year) from the private industry they are responsible for regulating. When this was reported to the head of the NIH, he initiated a requirement that honorariums be reported, and he reduced the maximum to $50,000.

I believe that any amount constitutes a conflict of interest. There are reports that prosecutions and regulatory actions by the FDA have gone down dramatically in number in recent years. Does this indicate that the industry regulated by the FDA is becoming more reliable, or is the FDA becoming more lax?

THE 2004 INFLUENZA VACCINE SHORTAGE

In the fall of 2004, practicing physicians were shocked by the government's announcement that we would be short of almost fifty million doses of flu vaccine.

---

30 A tissue sample is a biopsy or thin slice of flesh from the body of an animal or human. It's procured for the purpose of identifying a disease process or the effects of a medication or other treatment process.

Influenza kills thousands of people in the United States each year, especially among the infirm and elderly. The CDC directed all caregivers to limit the flu vaccination to that target population who needed it most.

How could such an enormous shortage happen? The news media informed us that one of the companies manufacturing the vaccine was having problems with bacterial contamination of the products from which the vaccine was made. The FDA is responsible for oversight of vaccine manufacturing facilities. They allegedly knew about the bacterial contamination problem as early as June 2003, yet took "less aggressive action than its inspectors initially recommended."[31]

The Chiron Company accepted the responsibility for manufacturing fifty million doses of flu vaccine for the 2004 season. It has a facility in Emeryville, California, but chose to do the manufacturing in England. The British health regulators shut down that plant in October 2004 after determining the purity of the vaccine couldn't be guaranteed.[32] It was further revealed in these news reports that the FDA was slow to reveal its 2003 findings to Chiron and there was no communication between our FDA and British health regulators.

31 "Democrats Fault FDA, Chiron in Vaccine Shortage," *Wall Street Journal*, 18 November 2004.

32 "Flu Vaccine Problems Run Deep," *Los Angeles Times*, 18 November 2004; "Objectives of JAMA," *JAMA*, 289 no. 1 (2003), 101.

Before I became a physician, I worked in public health for almost ten years. As an inspector, my mission was clear, protecting the public's health. We also recognized a need to be as helpful as we could and assist the industry we were regulating so they could achieve the goals we expected. The government paid us, not the industry we were regulating.

When I became a physician, I trusted the NIH and the FDA followed those same principles. Apparently, I was wrong!

ALTERNATIVE MEDICINE, NOT ALWAYS A GOOD ALTERNATIVE.

EVIDENCE-BASED MEDICINE AND TREATMENT

Science has always required that its proponents have a format in which to publish the information they have gathered so other scientists can review, criticize, or build on it. In its January 2003 issue, the peer-reviewed *Journal of the American Medical Association* describes what it expects from its authors.[33] This is how information that is necessary to the understanding of the benefits and risks of medicines is obtained and how the prescribers of these medications are educated in their use. If the prescribers and users of medicines are aware of the risks as well as the benefits of the substances being prescribed, then the greatest good can be achieved at the smallest risk.

Proponents of complementary and alternative medicine (CAM) have criticized accepted medical practice. In my opinion, CAM is often neither complementary, alternative, nor medicine. In the many years during which evidence-based medical research has been done, some treatment modalities that were considered alternative in the past were scientifically proven to be worthwhile. Those treatments have now

33 "Objectives of JAMA," *JAMA*, 289 no. 1 (2003), 101.

been accepted into the fold of traditional, evidence-based medicine. Other complementary and alternative products and treatments that have failed the tests of evidence-based science must remain as unproved modalities of care until scientific study has demonstrated their worth.

PAGING DR. FLEXNER

The practitioners of CAM rely on testimony as the only evidence they require to prove usefulness. They have amassed a large body of literature that they regard as peer reviewed and proof of efficacy. They have convinced Congress to create the National Center for Complementary and Alternative Medicine in the NIH. Congress has funded that agency with millions of dollars to study the worth of these treatments, many of which have already failed testing by excellent double-blind, peer-reviewed studies. The advocates of CAM are now on the staffs of some medical schools, teaching future doctors about alternative medicine and treatment.

The Dietary Supplement Health and Education Act of 1994 (DSHEA) has exempted many alternative products from regulation by the FDA. As a scientist and physician trained in evidence-based medicine, I realize the time has come for another Abraham Flexner. Dr. Flexner, working with support of the Carnegie Foundation for the advancement of teaching during the first decade of the twentieth century, surveyed all of the one hundred fifty-five medical schools that were then operating in the United States and Canada. His findings, published in 1910, resulted in the closing of the worst of the schools and led to the establishment of higher standards for medical education.

I am not implying that our medical schools aren't of high quality. I am hopeful that the discussion of CAM in some of our medical schools will be labeled as unproven modalities of care until they pass the tests of scientific proof.

ALTERATIVE TREATMENT IS OFTEN COSTLY AND OFTEN USELESS

During a recent two-week ocean cruise, one of our party signed up for the gym and exercise program. For an additional $450, she was offered pills that would help her lose weight while on the ship. The contents of the pills were not identified. Even the most powerful prescription weight control medications would not achieve a significant weight loss in two weeks, especially on a cruise ship offering unlimited amounts of food. If the pills were prescription weight control medicines, why was an exercise therapist offering them to passengers without a doctor's prior history and physical examination? If the offered pills were not prescription medicines, were they nonprescription alternatives that could cause significant weight loss in two weeks? I doubt it! Needless to say, our companion decided to forgo the entire program.

The promoters who sell CAM products to the public imply testimonials are equal to scientific proof. They are not! This is a free country, and individuals can choose as they wish, but the public needs more help when it comes to separating the science from the testimonials. Medical students should be trained to provide that help when they become practicing physicians. Medical schools should address the issue of alternative medical care, not as an evidence-based method of treatment, but as a modality of care that carefully evaluated evidence and scientific fact has not validated yet.

The next time you are urged to buy a product that claims to be natural and harmless or natural and safe, think twice. If a claim sounds too good to be true, it usually is. Nonprescription medicines or substances labeled as "natural" and "harmless" are often neither natural nor harmless. Let the buyer beware!

HIGH TEST? IRRADIATED? USE LESS?

After graduating from UCLA in 1949, I worked as a sanitarian (public health inspector) for health departments in California. One of the duties of a local health department sanitarian is to enforce the California Restaurant Act. It was then that I discovered some companies that supply products to restaurants, hotels, bars, and so forth sometimes misled and cheated the purchasers.

The California Restaurant Act required that restaurants sanitize (disinfect) all utensils that the public used in order to prevent the transfer of infections. This process could be accomplished with very hot water, a chlorine rinse, or a quaternary ammonium compound disinfectant. That requirement still exists.

A friend from college worked in the same health department, and we saw a lot of each other at work and socially. We noticed some of the companies that sold disinfecting products diluted their products so heavily with cheap, inert materials that the sanitizing solutions prepared with these products were far too dilute to disinfect anything. In spite of this, they were always labeled with words such as "industrial strength" and "full-strength," implying a small quantity went a long way.

In an effort to demonstrate this misrepresentation to our food service clients, we decided to invent a similar product that was entirely worthless. We called it "high test, irradiated, use less."

"Irradiated" was a powerful word in those days of the Cold War and implied great energy. Our product was irradiated when exposed to sunlight, a process that added no value to the substance, but certainly sounded potent. "High test" suggested the product was of great strength and had successfully passed rigorous testing. We assumed testing the material on the nineteenth floor of the city hall, where our health department's offices were, could be regarded as a version of a "high test." "Use less" implied one would need a smaller amount of the product to prepare a legally strong sanitizing solution. Actually, the word we were lampooning was "useless!"

Obviously, we never intended to market this product. It was a spoof of some of the so-called disinfecting products that the food service community, which we were responsible for overseeing, was then using. I strongly suspect that some establishments would have bought our fictitious product if it had been available.

PROFITS AS THE DRIVING FORCE

I tell this story to illustrate that, more than fifty years ago, I realized that industry too often puts profit and false claims ahead of the public's health. They still do! Many companies that sell vitamins, herbs, and health nostrums make false and unfounded claims in order to promote their products.

To make things worse, the FDA is virtually helpless to do anything about it because of the Hatch/Richardson Act. That job is left to the Federal Trade Commission (FTC), an agency that frequently is unable to do anything about unfounded claims.

Many companies that market herbs, vitamins, and natural remedies often make claims for efficacy that are untrue, but they are not required to reveal adverse effects. The pharmaceutical industry sometimes fails to report adverse incidents they are aware of, although the FDA regulations require they must.

It is important that a prescribing doctor should be made aware of possible adverse reactions that a drug might cause. This information must be described in the product brochure literature. There, it can be reviewed before prescribing the medicine. Obviously, this information could be a deterrent to prescribing the drug in question and would result in a loss of sales.

The entire purpose of reporting adverse reactions is patient protection. An industry that manufactures and sells medicines must be ever-aware that the very existence of the industry depends on patient safety. That is why this industry was once known as the "ethical drug industry."

I must commend the vast majority of the pharmaceutical industry for doing their best to obey this reporting requirement. I cannot say the same about alternative, complementary, and natural medicine promoters. There is little reliable or scientific evidence about either negative or positive effects, but that doesn't stop them from making positive proclamations and being silent about potentially serious negative effects that could result from the use of their product. Even if the product is harmless, it could divert the patient from the use of an effective, proven treatment.

Medical doctors rarely recommend alternative and complementary methods of treatment. However, doctors sometimes prescribe yet-to-be-proven treatments, especially for patients who are terminally ill and desperate.

POISON, CUT, AND BURN

A physician practicing in the Los Angeles area, though he is trained in traditional medicine, decided mainstream doctors "poison, cut and burn" so he became a practitioner of complementary and alternative medicine. One of my patients went to him with her mother, an elderly woman who was becoming increasingly lethargic. He decided her mother was vitamin deficient and prescribed mega doses of multivitamins.

The vitamin regimen failed to improve mother's status. In fact, her condition worsened. The patient was brought to me. After obtaining a short history and doing a brief examination, third-year medical students could have made the diagnosis. She wasn't vitamin deficient. My impression was that she had myxedema, caused by thyroid hormone deficiency.

I confirmed this impression by ordering thyroid function tests that validated the diagnosis. I then placed her on a regimen of thyroid medication. In a few weeks, she was back to her former self. From her alternative medicine doctor's viewpoint, as well as the title of this book, I poisoned her, but she got better. Thyroid medicine can indeed be dangerous when used in excessive dosage, but, when used at therapeutic levels, the results are sometimes miraculous, as they were in this case.

Even relatively innocuous agents, such as vitamins, are capable of causing harm, if they divert patients from a medicine or treatment that can help them to regain their health.

MORE TROUBLE FOR THIS FAMILY

A few months later, this patient's daughter came to me, complaining she was suffering from left flank pain. I did a urinalysis and found microscopic amounts of blood in her urine. Suspecting a kidney stone, I sent her for an ultrasonic study of the kidneys and ureters (the tubes that transmit the urine from the kidneys to the bladder). There was no evidence of stones, but a mass was seen in the left kidney. Further studies revealed nothing else, although they did confirm the kidney mass. It was likely to be malignant.

When I told her she could have cancer and might need surgery, the patient told me that the diagnosis had to be wrong because she was taking shark cartilage. The same doctor who missed her mother's myxedema had prescribed the shark cartilage. He had told her that she should take shark cartilage because sharks don't get cancer. (They do, according to marine biologists, who should know.)

I referred her to the urologist, who had cared for me when I had my prostate surgery. He immediately hospitalized her. During the subsequent surgery, he removed a large tumor that the pathologist diagnosed as a renal cell carcinoma (kidney cancer). The surgeon had cut my patient and burned her by cauterizing blood vessels to control bleeding. I was about to refer her to an oncologist who would poison her with cancer-killing chemicals.

Kidney cancers are notorious for their tendency to spread to other parts of the body (metastasize), but her studies did not reveal any evidence of this at the time of her surgery. Repeat studies were questionable. One of the radiologists carefully studied her X-rays and suspected early signs of cancer were in her lungs (metastasis). The patient was a nurse by profession and had been reading about renal cell carcinoma. When she heard about our concerns, she said, "I'm dead!"

Her self-prophecy was accurate. The tumor grew rapidly and soon clearly revealed itself in her lungs. Her oncologist honored her request for palliative care only. She was hospitalized and died quietly and without discomfort because she was willing to use the cancer specialist's prescripted poisons. The poisons he gave her were sedatives and analgesics, including morphine, to ease her pain.

I believe that, during the years of my medical practice, I provided my patients with a complete spectrum of medical services. When I perceived my patients had a medical problem beyond my own expertise, I promptly referred them to the most qualified specialist I knew about.

One patient desperately needed heart surgery in the early days of that procedure. For religious reasons, she wanted it done without the use of blood. I referred her to Dr. Denton Cooley, a heart surgeon in Texas who was considered to be among the best in the world. He graciously accepted her and successfully did her heart surgery without the use of blood or blood products.

NATURAL AND HARMLESS

Recently, the FDA analyzed a nonprescription medicine that was reported to correct erectile dysfunction. It was found to contain sildenafil, the same generic, prescription-controlled ingredient that makes Viagra work. This ingredient was not mentioned on the label of the OTC product that was being sold as natural. Sildenafil is neither natural nor harmless. OTC erectile dysfunction medications must not contain active ingredients that would require a prescription. That's illegal! The other truth is that OTC products that claim erectile dysfunction treatment don't contain any ingredient that is definitely proven to treat erectile dysfunction. They probably rely on the placebo effect.

The FDA product brochure for Viagra (sildenafil) warns patients who are using an anti-angina medicine containing nitrites (nitroglycerine) that sildenafil can induce a sudden blood pressure drop that could cause fainting, and rarely, death. The product brochure also describes the possibility of blue vision, which is considered to be more annoying than harmful. In addition, blindness, a rare side effect, has recently been reported due to the use of this family of medicines. But there was no warning on the so-called natural erectile-enhancing products. This is not an isolated example of misbranding and misrepresentation that goes on in the OTC market.

Some OTC weight-loss products have been found to contain ephedra or ephedra-like substances that are now banned in both the United States and Canada, but there was no statement on the label or in any accompanying information that the product contained an ephedra-like substance. A federal judge ruled the FDA has not proved that low doses of ephedra in OTC preparations are harmful. So the FDA had no control over the OTC preparations containing ten milligrams or less of this active ingredient. Since then, the FDA has successfully appealed and reversed the judge's decision.

THE NATURAL HERB THAT PROBABLY HAS CAUSED THE MOST GRIEF

I'd be remiss if I didn't discuss the herb that has caused more human grief than any other in history, tobacco. It certainly qualifies as natural, but we'll all agree that it's far from harmless. Aside from its medical issues, tobacco has caused numerous fires, stained clothing, burned holes in fabrics, smoke damage, and so forth. The medical hazards were suspected as early as the nineteenth century when cigarettes were called "coffin nails" and, more recently, "cancer sticks." The surgeon general proclaimed that secondhand cigarette smoke is harmful to people exposed to it.

I have always considered tobacco to be an unpleasant substance. When I joined the navy at age seventeen in 1944, the military forces were being sold cigarettes that were offered at fifty cents a carton or five cents a pack. I was the only one in my platoon who didn't smoke. I gave away my ration. I tolerated a lot of ribbing because I didn't smoke. When my platoon mates asked me why, I asked them to tell me which animal in nature runs toward smoke. The only time that strategy failed was when one of my young patients told me that the rhinoceros runs toward the smoke in order to stamp out the fire. He knew that because he had seen it on a TV cartoon show.

In the early 1950s, the radio program *Dragnet* was a dramatization of the Los Angeles Police Department's detective work. A cigarette company sponsored it. Each episode aired a running report from a prominent doctor, stating the advertised cigarette was found to cause "no damage to the throat, nose, and sinuses." The commercial was conspicuous in its failure to mention the lungs or any other organ system. In the years I have been a physician, I have seen patients with cancer in the bladder and lungs attributed to cigarette smoking and mouth and tongue cancer due to cigars and chewing tobacco.

THE POWER OF ADDICTION

When I was in training at Los Angeles County General Hospital, I saw a patient who was afflicted with arteriosclerosis obliterans, a disease that literally causes the peripheral arteries to scar down to such narrow channels that the tissues being nurtured by these vessels die. Smoking accelerates the deterioration. This patient's fingers were so withered and deteriorated by his disease that he couldn't hold anything. He was a smoker who was so addicted to cigarettes that he wore a wrist bracelet equipped with a clip to hold his cigarette.

I had been in practice a little over a year when I hospitalized a patient with emphysema (a form of severe lung disease). The patient was in serious respiratory distress. He was on oxygen and receiving medications to open his bronchial airways, yet he insisted on continuing his smoking. I explained we couldn't give him oxygen while he smoked. He said he had to have his cigarettes and insisted the nurse must remove the oxygen tank from his room so he could smoke.

Although smoking was allowed in the hospitals in those days, the situation became so intolerable that I had to discharge him to his home. He agreed to sign out against medical advice, which relieved the hospital of responsibility for the consequences of his premature discharge. Within a few weeks, he died of his lung disease. On his death certificate, I wrote "death due to severe chronic lung disease, due to cigarette smoking."

Shortly thereafter, I received a call from a local radio talk show host who interviewed me on the air, asking why I had signed the underlying cause of death due to cigarettes. I suspect somebody at the Registrar of Death Certificates office tipped off the host of the talk show about the death certificate I had sent in. This was several years before the release of the surgeon general's report stating that cigarettes may be harmful to your health. Since then, I have treated hundreds of patients harmed by tobacco.

WHO GETS THE BLAME?

A recent case reminded me of a malpractice trial that I read about in one of the medical journals. The trial was about a patient who died from pelvic cancer. The defendant physician was being sued because he failed to diagnose the cancer. He told his malpractice insurer that he had an excellent defense. The decedent had been repeatedly encouraged to submit to a pelvic examination and Pap smear, which she repeatedly refused. It was only when her daughter persuaded her mother to have the examination done by her own doctor that the cancer was discovered. The defense lost because the court ruled the doctor wasn't persuasive enough in his efforts to convince the patient to agree to have a pelvic examination.

Shortly after reading about this decision, the daughter of one of my patients came to see me about her chest congestion and cough. After examining her, I was alarmed enough to hospitalize her. She was a smoker. During the many previous visits to my office with her mother, who was also my patient, I had repeatedly told her to quit smoking. Her hospital studies revealed multiple lesions in her lungs. The subsequent bronchoscopy demonstrated cancer cells. I called an oncologist into consultation, and she was immediately started on aggressive chemotherapy.

I had known this patient for a long time because I had taken care of her elderly mother until she died. The patient was a wonderful human being. I regarded her as a friend as well as a patient. In spite of every therapy, she was dying, and she knew it. At her bedside one day, I was lamenting out loud that I should have absolutely insisted she quit smoking. She responded, "You didn't put the cigarettes in my mouth." But, even if I had persuaded her to quit, she might have gotten cancer anyway. Tobacco is a poison!

ANOTHER SMOKY ISSUE

Smoking anything is probably deleterious, so, to be consistent, I must conclude that smoking marijuana or anything else is not good for you. Marijuana is also used as medicine. By now, I hope you are convinced that all medicines are poison. I have prescribed the equivalent of the active ingredient in marijuana as a prescription medicine. That medicine is an FDA-approved drug known as Marinol or Dronabinol. It's not a smoke, but it's useful for relieving nausea in terminally ill cancer patients. I have never prescribed smoking marijuana under any circumstances, although it's now legal to do so for medical purposes in many states, including California, where I practiced medicine.

The active ingredient in marijuana is cannabis, which does have sedative effects. As with any sedative, its effects should be respected. Because I have personally never used a cannabis-containing substance myself, I cannot describe its effect first-hand. Logic, as well as experience with various inhaled medications, tells me that inhaled material doesn't work very differently on the body than the injected material.

Opinion in our country is divided on the subject of medical marijuana. I have always suspected that a portion of people who claim they support medicinal smoking of marijuana are actually supporting its recreational use. But, if I have a patient who is terminally ill and believes marijuana will help to relieve his or her suffering, how can I say I won't prescribe it?

Although the voters in seventeen states have already approved the legal use of medical marijuana in their respective jurisdictions, at the time this was written, the federal law still considered its use as unlawful. Federal enforcement authorities have now decided not to prosecute anyone who grows, sells, or uses it for medicinal purposes.

The next time you are urged to buy a product that claims to be natural and harmless or natural and safe, think twice. If a claim sounds too good to be true, it usually is. Medicines or substances labeled "natural" and "harmless" are often neither natural nor harmless. Let the buyer beware!

GINKGO BILOBA AND OTHER NONPRESCRIPTION CURES

I trained and worked as a public health sanitarian and subsequently as a sanitary engineer in California before I went to medical school to become a doctor. One of the locations on my inspection route was a bar that had existed since the Jack London days. A free lunch setup was at this bar. You could select a hard-boiled egg or pickled pig's feet, but you had to buy a beer or a shot of whiskey first so the free lunch wasn't really free.

Recently, one of my patients asked if a new medicine I had prescribed for her had any side effects. "All medicines have side effects," I responded. "There is no free lunch!"

Even water and air can be toxic in certain circumstances. Drinking too much water can wash vital chemicals, such as sodium and potassium, out of your body. That can cause weakness and bodily malfunctions. Breathing too rapidly can blow away essential levels of carbon dioxide and cause a person to be light-headed and even faint. The antidote is to breathe into a paper bag and restore the necessary carbon dioxide level.

Many people agree prescription medicines can be poisonous, but anything labeled "natural" is not. While many natural substances are relatively harmless, some contain dangerous components. For example, everyone knows about poisonous mushrooms and toadstools, but most people are unable to determine which mushrooms are safe to eat. There are harmless snakes and poisonous snakes.

The British navy was correct when it supplied all of its ships with limes for the crews to prevent scurvy. Actually, vitamin C in the lime prevented the disease. Now, science accepts the use of vitamin C to prevent scurvy as a proven fact.

Linus Pauling, a Nobel Prize-winning chemist, believed mega doses of vitamin C would cure the common cold. Studies have disproved this, but millions of people still use vitamin C for this purpose. Mega doses of vitamin C are not entirely harmless. They can precipitate diarrhea and even disrupt the normal chemical balance of the body. Just because a little is good, a lot may not necessarily be better.

SOME NATURAL SUBSTANCES THAT YIELD MEDICINES

Many prescription medicines are actually derived from natural substances. Digitalis, a heart medicine, is derived from the foxglove plant. Warfarin is a blood thinner made from a substance found in spoiled hay. Quinine is an antimalarial drug made from the bark of a tree.

Hippocrates is said to have prescribed the bark of the willow tree steeped in boiling water to make a tea that reduced fever and relieved pain. The substance in willow bark that imparts these effects is essentially similar to aspirin.

I could name many others, but these are some examples. There are natural substances and vitamins that are dangerous and poisonous, yet they are being advertised and sold to the public without a prescription. Vitamin D and calcium tablets sound innocuous enough. Millions of postmenopausal women whose bones are weakened by the loss of calcium are taking these substances at the suggestion of their doctors. Millions of infants are taking multivitamins, but excessive dosage can be harmful.

The FDA has no control or oversight of the herb and nutritional market because this industry has persuaded Congress to make laws that exempt them from FDA controls. As a physician trained in public health, I was under the impression that one of the duties of the FDA was to protect the public from dangerous substances and false claims of efficacy. The Hatch/Richardson Dietary Supplement Health and Education Act (DSHEA) of

1994, however, protects the public's right to buy and consume any vitamin or herb they want.

The act's definition of a dietary supplement is so broad that the FDA's mandate to protect the public from false claims by the purveyors of this class of nonprescription products is thwarted. The act defines a "dietary ingredient" as a substance that may include "vitamins, minerals, herbs, or other botanical, amino acids, and substances such as enzymes, organ tissues, glandular, and metabolic."

The act does have rules against making false or misleading claims, but, except in the case of a new dietary ingredient, the marketing firm "does not have to provide the FDA with the evidence that it relies on to substantiate safety or effectiveness" before or after it markets its products. I view this as manufacturer protectionism, not consumer protectionism.

AN HERBAL SUBSTANCE WORTHY OF DISCUSSION

Ginkgo biloba is a plant derivative that is promoted by herbologists and others who encourage alternative medicines. They claim this herb is useful for the treatment of numerous problems, including memory deficits, depression, dizziness, ringing in the ears, reduced blood circulation to the extremities, and other problems often attributed to vascular insufficiency. The leaf of the plant is said to contain many pharmacologically active substances that are thought to act together in the whole leaf extract but do not show the same activity individually.

Until recently, I was unaware of any information in the medical literature that reported scientifically proven benefits from using it. However, recent studies by UCLA suggest that Ginkgo biloba "may protect memory in older patients."[34] This study revealed several risk factors such as strokes and bleeding-related complications. If the benefits prove to outweigh the risks, Ginkgo biloba extracts might be added to the list of useful medicines, but it needs further evaluation before that becomes a fact.

If Ginkgo biloba is really as effective as its proponents say it is, I would anticipate that a few users would have minimal benefits, but most people would report good to wonderful benefits from Ginkgo biloba in the conditions it is expected to help. This statistic should slant the curve strongly to the "effective" side when graphed. But I have seen several reports in the evidence-based literature that failed to support the anecdotes declaring the great benefits of Ginkgo biloba.[35]

---

34 Mary Hardy, "UCLA Division of Geriatrics," August 2008.

35 P.R. Solomon, et al., "Ginkgo for Memory Enhancement: A Randomized Controlled Study," *JAMA*, 288 no. 7 (2002), 835–840.

I'm reminded of what my statistics professor at UCLA told us when we were studying the public's health trends. She said, "Statistics never lie, but liars compile statistics." She also illustrated the bell-shaped curves and their pictorial value in graphing statistics.

The bell shaped curve is a way of graphing statistical information. An epidemic of Flu would graph as follows: The curve illustrated in Figure 1 depicts a Flu epidemic during which most patients are only moderately ill. Figure 2 is slanting to the left, indicating that most people who caught the flu virus had no symptoms, or were only mildly ill. Figure 3 plots a severe epidemic, where most people were moderately or severely ill and a few even died.

THE BELL-SHAPED CURVES

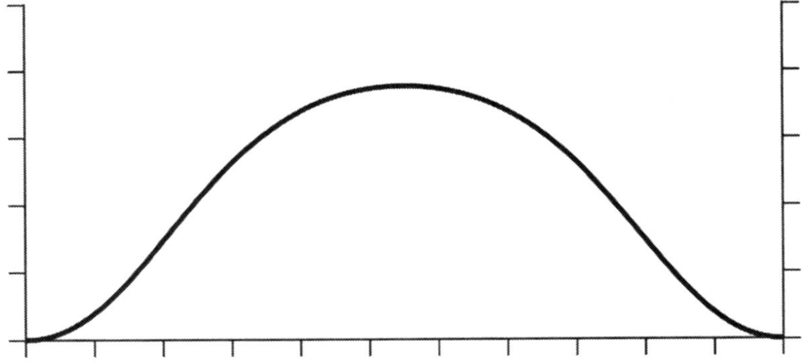

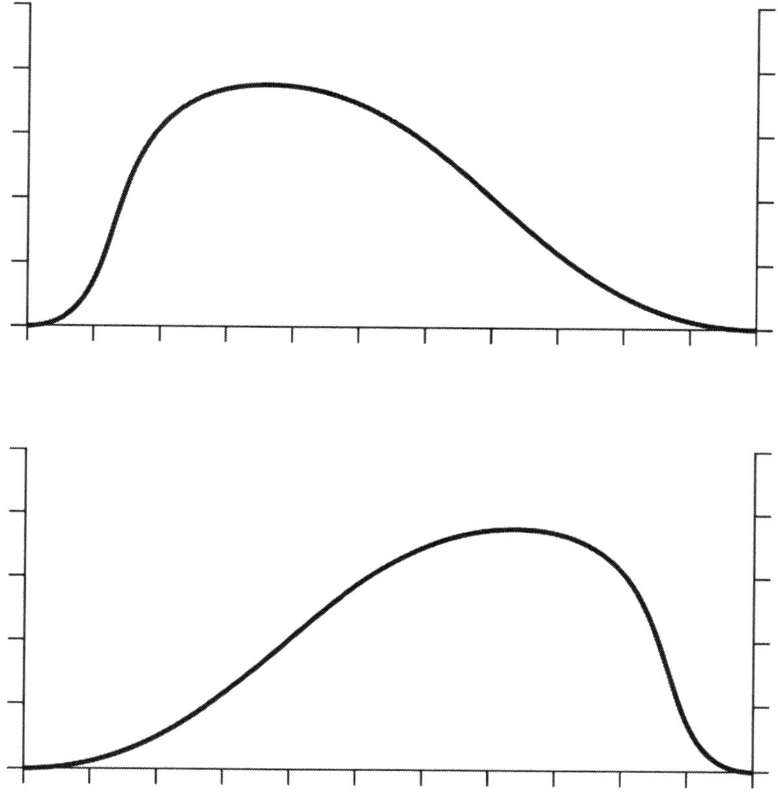

WATCH OUT FOR STATISTICS

This discussion reminds me of a story my accountant related to me. He told me that a corporation sent an annual statement to its shareholders stating there had been a 20 percent improvement in profits since the prior year. The corporation subsequently told its employees union that there had only been a one percent increase in profits compared to the prior year. Both statements were true. How could that be? The prior year's profit was 4 percent of gross; the current year's profit was 5 percent of gross. My accountant was right. Do the math!

DISCOVERING VALUE IN UNEXPECTED PLACES

In spite of what my patients tell me about their negative experiences with Ginkgo biloba, I do believe there are herbs and chemicals of significant value yet to be welcomed into the realm of scientific medicine. When I was a graduate student at UCLA in 1949, my chemistry professor assigned me a project. The object was to find a use for the substance glucosamine.

First, I had to go to the university library catacombs to look up and laboriously translate the German chemical literature, where much of the glucosamine chemistry had already been reported. Then I had to make glucosamine in the laboratory. The exoskeletons of crustaceans are constructed of a glucosamine polymer, scientifically known as chitin, infiltrated with calcium to harden it.

I collected lobster shells from the local expensive restaurants that served lobster dinners. Then I removed the calcium by soaking the lobster shells in hydrochloric acid. With the calcium removed, what remained was the tough, flexible, plastic-like chitinous shell. My goal was to depolymerize the chitin into the glucosamine molecule. I was then planning to repolymerize the glucosamine back into a durable plastic that could have commercial value. I never succeeded or suspected that, fifty years later, glucosamine would become a popular arthritis remedy. I still have remnants of that glucosamine experiment stored in my garage. My wife complains I never throw anything away.

MEDICAL FRAUD AND OTHER SHENANIGANS

When I was working at the California State Health Department in the early 1950s, I became aware that our department was investigating medical and health fraud. We had amassed a gallery of phony devices confiscated from so-called medical practitioners. Many were chiropractors.

One such device was confiscated from a woman chiropractor in Hollywood who practiced remote healing. One of her patients had contacted us because he had doubts regarding the medical treatment she was giving to him. She told him she had invented a medical device that could do remote healing. When the patient called in sick, she would insert the patient's blood, which she had stored for such an eventuality, into the device for treatment. That action was supposed to cure the patient's illness, no matter how far away he might actually be physically.

Over fifty years later, the claim of remote healing may seem outlandish, but, after the attack on the World Trade Center, Wayne Jonas and Pat Linton published a commentary piece stating that our military could prevent future terrorists attacks by means of remote viewing.[36] Remote viewing is a psychic technique that permits people who claim to have such an ability to see events that are now occurring thousands of miles away or will happen in the future.

Our military authorities studied remote viewing years ago, but they were never able to validate the process, much less find any verifiable information at all by using the technique. In these experiments, remote viewers were unable to locate our own warships. They were unsuccessful even though the military personnel they were working with knew of the exact location of the warships the remote viewers were seeking. They'd have been better off if they were mind readers. Maybe our military experts should hire mind readers to interrogate spies. Then again, maybe not!

When Groucho Marx's quiz show was on television years ago, one of his contestants claimed she was a mind reader. Nevertheless, she failed to guess the secret word and win $100, even though Groucho's television staff

---

36 Linton and Jonas, "Commentary," *Honolulu Advertiser*, 25 August 2002.

knew what it was and were waiting for her to say it so they could release a duck marionette from the ceiling with a card in its mouth bearing the secret word. One of my friends asked why a psychic who meets you for the first time asks for your name instead of spontaneously using it.

If remote viewing were possible, why didn't some remote viewer detect the terrorists' plan to fly commercial airplanes into the World Trade Center and warn the authorities? For that matter, why didn't all the psychics in the world, who claim to foresee almost everything, see the inevitable and horrendous attack and warn us?

Linton and Jonas also proposed that alternative medical modalities, such as acupuncture and homeopathy, be used for the wounded in military operations, including on the battlefield itself. Somehow, I cannot believe the role of the medic will ever be to crawl, under hostile fire, to the side of a wounded soldier and insert acupuncture needles into his body to relieve his pain or administer homeopathic solutions to heal his wounds and prevent infection.

DETOXIFICATION PROCEDURES

When I first went into medical practice, high colonic enemas were still popular and being recommended by some medical practitioners. The purpose of this procedure was to cleanse the colon of toxins and other substances considered to be bad for one's health. Years ago, I joined an associate who had recently moved into a medical office that a doctor who did high colonics had previously occupied. The apparatus for this procedure consisted of an enema-administering device and glass tubing through which the back washings flowed from the colon. The glass tubing was employed to show the patient the toxic wastes and other evil substances that were being removed from his or her bowels. My partner and I decided to immediately remove the apparatus from our office! High colonics are no longer popular as a detoxifier. I doubt they ever really detoxified anything, although an impacted or severely constipated patient can sometimes benefit from an enema.

Colonoscopy is now the accepted procedure recommended for finding cancerous growths of the colon in people who are at risk for this disease. This procedure does require thorough bowel cleansing. However, the cleansing wastes no longer flow though a glass tubing for the patient to see, although there is a monitor screen to watch if a person is awake enough during the colonoscopy procedure. In view of the past use of the glass tubing, I suppose we have to conclude that what goes around comes around.

DEATH BY DIETARY SUPPLEMENTS

Recently, a patient suffering from macular degeneration (deterioration of the nerve ending in the eyeball that makes it possible to see) showed me a medicine she bought from a salesman who claimed the product would help her visual problems. The fact is that, until recently, standard science could do almost nothing for macular degeneration. Canadian research developed a dye/laser treatment that seems to help one type of macular degeneration. But there are two types, and medical science has yet to discover how to control the other type. This leaves things wide open for the dietary supplement regimens.

The salesman was pitching a concoction of numerous vitamins, minerals, and herbs that a company calling itself the Science-Based Company was marketing. I seriously doubt the company did any valid scientific research at all. If they did, I'd welcome reading about that research in an evidence-based medical journal. Good evidence would persuade me to change my opinion. Anyone trained in science studies the evidence before arriving at a conclusion. That's why the name "Science-Based Company" sounds so impressive.

The use of this particular name to imply their product is based on scientific testing reminds me of the days when Japanese products were cheaply and poorly made. A Japanese manufacturer based itself in a location in Japan named Usa. I'm uncertain that such a place actually existed, but I recently heard someone else mention Usa. Their products were labeled "made in USA," obviously implying they were made in the United States and not in Japan, where they were actually manufactured. "Made in Japan" now implies quality and integrity, often superior to products made in the United States. The evidence is there to prove it.

I did an Internet search for Science-Based Company. I was amazed at the amount of material I found. I also found references to dietary regimens and something called "silent inflammation." Allegedly, a condition caused by silent inflammation fails to respond to any known anti-inflammatories and does not reveal itself to any scientific methods I am aware of or trained in. I searched through my medical dictionary and textbooks and found no reference to silent inflammation. I wondered if the people who have written about these things have created a new science of their own.

One of my colleagues was aware of silent inflammation. Although he agreed that contemporary medical educators do not discuss silent inflammation, his impression is that there may be such an entity. He also believes it may eventually become an accepted entity of evidence-based science.

SHOULD DIETARY SUPPLEMENTS BE REGULATED?

A paper, "Death by Dietary Supplement," reported thousands of adverse reactions and many deaths attributed to dietary supplements, which the FDA recorded until 1998 when they stopped monitoring them.[37] The authors suggested a voluntary organization, such as Underwriters Laboratory or Good Housekeeping, regulate the industry so a seal of approval would offer assurance the supplement is at least safe and harmless, if not actually useful.

There is a powerful need for humans to believe and a mighty ability to convince themselves that this belief is correct. I'm not referring to religion, though that is a good example. Humankind has developed over two thousand religions, each viewed by its proponents as the one true belief. I'm referring to the fervor with which a

37 Miller and Longton, "Death by Dietary Supplement," *Hoover Institute Publications* (November 2000).

person believes that something works. This is probably due to the placebo effect.

DO VITAMINS AND STEROIDS PROVIDE A COMPETITIVE EDGE?

Ergonomic aids are substances that enhance energy production, use, or recovery. Athletes believe that use of these substances will give them a competitive advantage. Surveys have reported that approximately half of the general population take supplements. Other surveys have shown that 76 percent of college athletes and 100 percent of bodybuilders take supplements.

The author of this study reviewed the research on numerous ergonomic substances. He summarized the action and observed benefits (or lack thereof), side effects, and legality in sports. Substances such as anabolic steroids were effective in producing the desired results, but had significant dangers. They are illegal for use in competition. Research found that androstenedione, a steroid first reported to be used by home run hitter Mark McGwire and many other athletes, had limited or no benefits. It may have significant side effects. The NCAA and the International Olympic Committee have banned it. Barry Bonds, who broke the all-time home run record, was also accused of using steroids. He denied this.[38] However, many well-known athletes have admitted using what are known as "enhancing drugs."

In 2004, the drug DHEA (dehydroepiandrosterone) escaped the ban due to the actions of Senator Orrin G. Hatch of Utah, who co-authored DSHEA, the Dietary Supplement Health and Education Act. Utah is where many dietary supplements are produced. His son, Scott Hatch, was (and may still be) a lobbyist for the National Nutritional Foods Association and has represented firms that sell DHEA. Senator Hatch argued DHEA must be legal and available as an anti-aging pill.[39] There is no scientific proof that DHEA can prevent aging. Furthermore, such a study would take many years to complete and would require a statistically significant number of participants, unbiased scientists, patients taking placebos, and valid methods of measuring aging.

The widely used B vitamins were found to have no benefit unless there is a preexisting deficiency. This is unlikely in an athlete. Other than producing a vitamin-rich urine, they probably have no side effects. They are legal in competition. Yet, if an athlete believes a supplement works, no amount of scientific proof that it doesn't work will dissuade its use.

---

38 This accusation was not verified at the time this was written.

39 Kornblut and Wilson, *New York Times*, 17 April 2005.

WHAT ELSE DON'T VITAMINS CURE?

The experience with the general population is similar. A double-blind study of cold remedies at a well-known university demonstrated this. Actor Alan Alda documented this study on his popular public television show, *Scientific America Frontiers*. Each participant, including Mr. Alda, was given a cold by spraying rhinovirus into the nose. The cold was then treated with various substances, including vitamin C and zinc. The subjects couldn't believe their favorite cold remedy worked no better than a placebo.

Studies showed that populations with high homocysteine blood levels were at greater risk of strokes and heart attacks. It was found the B vitamins (folic acid, B6, and B12) reduce the level of homocysteine. It was therefore generally accepted that this B vitamin regimen would reduce the risk of heart attacks and strokes. However, three recent studies have shown the B vitamin dietary supplementation is really not effective in benefiting or reversing advanced vascular disease.[40]

In the early years of my medical practice, I delivered babies and cared for many children. It was (and still is) standard medical practice to recommend a multivitamin supplement. The infant vitamin formula most often

40 "Studies Suggest B Vitamins Don't Prevent Heart Attacks," *New York Times*, 13 March 2006.

recommended contained vitamins A, B complex, C, and D. The prescription equivalent also contained fluoride for teeth. Years ago, nutritional scientists determined that vitamins A and D were toxic in excessive amounts so the producers of these formulas found it necessary to reduce the amount of those two ingredients to about two-thirds of the amount that these popular infant vitamins had previously contained. The revised formulas reached the marketplace accompanied by a fanfare of advertising claiming, "New Improved Formula! No Advance in Price!" Surprise! There was no advance in prices even though there were fewer ingredients in the new formula. The empty bottle and advertising campaign probably cost more than the vitamins!

Vitamins A and D are toxic in excessive amounts. Vitamin K can interfere with thinning of the blood in people who must take anticoagulants. Dietitians and university-trained nutritionists advocate the best way to get your vitamins is from the foods found in a balanced diet.

DOES EVERYONE NEED EXTRA VITAMINS?

Some nutritionists who sell herbs and vitamin supplements claim to have a doctor's degree in nutrition. Mail-order diploma mills are selling doctor degrees in nutrition. Dr. Victor Herbert, who had a degree in both medicine and law and did vitamin research years ago, once told us that both his dog and his cat had mail-order doctor's degrees in nutrition, which he had purchased from diploma mills.

I recommend *The Vitamin Pushers*, authored jointly by Dr. Herbert and Dr. Stephen Barrett, for much worthwhile information regarding vitamins.[41] Dr. Herbert is now deceased. Those of us who knew him miss his powerful voice against health fraud. Dr. Barrett is still publishing his energetic and enlightening Web site about medical dishonesty and health fraud at quackwatch.org.

An article regarding the pros and cons of taking vitamins appeared in the *Los Angeles Times*. It discusses double-blind, controlled studies involving as many as thirty-six thousand people. The article discussed the limited value of taking vitamins.[42]

Most Americans don't need to take vitamins because the food that our population consumes is readily available in large variety, and many of these foods are already fortified with vitamins. (Read the labels.) If you still feel you need to take vitamin supplements, take them in moderation.

---

41 *The Vitamin Pushers: How the Health Food Industry Is Selling America a Bill of Goods* (Prometheus Press, 1994).

42 Karen Kaplan, "Vitamins can only do so much," *Los Angeles Times*, 12 November 2008.

HOMEOPATHIC, CHIROPRACTIC, AND HOLISTIC MEDICINE

As a member of the board of NCAHF, I was asked to serve as an expert witness in a case against a chiropractor who owned a company that produced homeopathic products. I knew only one physician in the medical community where I practiced who used homeopathic drugs, and my role was to attest to that. With that one exception, every medical doctor I interviewed said he or she did not believe that homeopathic drugs worked, except perhaps as a placebo.

Homeopathy is based on a concept invented in the nineteenth century by the German physician, Dr. Samuel Hahnemann. He conjectured that if he treated a patient with minuscule quantities of a substance that at full strength caused similar symptoms as the illness, it would counter the symptoms and make the illness go away.

As prepared today, the harmful sustances are diluted serially and shaken with large quantities of pure water until there is essentially none of the original substance in the water. Homeopaths maintain the shaking and diluting process imprints the water molecules with new properties, even though only a few molecules of the active harmful substances are left in the resultant solution. This concoction is then used to treat the illness.

The practice flies in the face of the known principles of physics and medical science. Numerous evidence-based studies have failed to show benefits other than the placebo effect. As previously stated, placebos can have a beneficial effect early on, but they eventually prove to be of no value beyond that.

Before the trial started, the owner of the homeopathic product company approached one of my colleagues from NCAHF and asked why he was so against homeopathy. I then learned that the owner of the homeopathic products company was a chiropractor. At that point, I suddenly realized what was going on. Many of the customers and prescribers of homeopathic products are chiropractors. For years, chiropractors have been trying to obtain the right to prescribe medicines, but, to date, they have never been given the legal privilege to do so.

To get around this limitation and appear to be writing real prescription medicines, they would order homeopathic preparations in addition to the usual OTC vitamins and herbs. Now they could finally recommend substances that some people regard as prescription drugs, though they are actually nonprescription preparations. This adds a sense of legitimacy to their ability to treat disease beyond the use of chiropractic manipulation and massage.

As already stated, physicians believe homeopathic drugs are no more than placebos. So why worry about a bit of harmless pure water labeled as a medicine? This book has clearly reported that all medicines have side effects whose risks may sometimes outweigh their benefits. A homeopathic drug may make a patient feel better, even if it's the result of the placebo effect. As already indicated, many illnesses get better without treatment.

My concern is twofold. First, the patient may be getting nothing and believes he or she is getting something of benefit. Second, the patient may have an illness that needs medical treatment or may be contagious, and nothing curative is being done. The first is fraud; the second is dangerous. The patient has a right to know about such issues. The ancient rule of medicine advised by Hippocrates in his oath, "First do no harm," applies here.

WHAT IS CHIROPRACTIC?

D.D. Palmer invented chiropractic in 1895. He theorized that all disease is due to misalignment of the vertebrae (subluxations). The chiropractic manipulation of the spine allegedly corrects the misalignments, and the patient gets better. Manipulations may have an effect similar to massage. Massage therapy, an accepted method of treatment, is frequently prescribed for the relief of pain. It comes under the category of laying on of hands, and it is used to reduce painful muscle tightness and spasms. I believe chiropractic owes its benefit to the laying on of hands, not to the correction of the misalignments of the spine. Trained massage therapists can do everything a chiropractor can do and provide just as much relief. They don't regard themselves as doctors. Chiropractors call themselves doctors and imply they have all of the skills and abilities of a physician, yet, to this time, they have never been granted the medicine-prescribing approval, which they have vigorously sought.

I once watched a TV talk show that hosted a chiropractor, herbalist, other people who claimed to be healers, and one of the prominent professors of medicine from my medical school. The chiropractor claimed chiropractic school was longer and more comprehensive than traditional medical training and chiropractors are better and safer healers than graduates of traditional medical school training. The professor from my medical school was not permitted to interrupt, but I could see him writhe in disbelief at some of the statements that the moderator left unchallenged.

Although chiropractors are not permitted to write prescriptions, they have tried. In lieu of the ability to order prescription medicines, they prescribe liberally from the voluminous list of vitamins, herbs, and other OTC agents. Some of the NSAIDs that are now available without a prescription are excellent pain medicines. One of my patients told me she had received a supply of those medicines from the drawer of the chiropractor's desk at a time when all anti-inflammatory medications still required a prescription.

Although the chiropractor on the TV show was convinced his chiropractic training was better than the education that medical schools offered, doctors in the United States must document training at a quality medical school and teaching hospital. There, they see every manner of medical problem and are required to keep up their medical education throughout their years in practice.

WHAT IS HOLISTIC MEDICINE?

Some medical doctors advertise they practice holistic medicine. What is holistic medicine? They say, "We treat the whole patient." Actually, family practitioners are trained to treat the whole patient, but they must be realistic about their own limitations. Problems beyond a family practitioner's skills should be referred to a qualified consultant who has specialty training in areas of diagnosis and treatment where the family practitioner is lacking. This includes heart catheterization, neurosurgery, oncology, endocrinology, psychotherapy, neonatology, and other areas of expertise that comprise the whole patient but require special knowledge. No Board of Holistic Medicine tests the doctor's knowledge of his or her field of practice and requires he or she has passed a rigorous, daylong recertification test every six years. The Board of Family Practice and other medical specialty boards do have that requirement.

Family practitioners do not need to label themselves as holistic. It's redundant. I believe that, when doctors label themselves as holists, it implies to the patient and the world that the holistic doctor is qualified to use diagnostic and treatment methods that a traditional doctor does not have the skill or knowledge to utilize. Those additional modalities are often beyond evidence-based medical practices. A holistic doctor often utilizes CAM. The many reasons for my reluctance to adopt these practices are discussed everywhere in this book.

KNOW YOUR LIMITS

I have a firm policy of only referring my patients to specialists I would trust to care for my family and myself. As a senior citizen, whose own health has failed on several occasions, I have had plenty of opportunity to determine who the best doctors are. I do not use alternative or complementary treatments unless they are thoroughly and scientifically studied and have clearly demonstrated they are worthwhile. But, when that process has proven them to be worthy, they are no longer regarded as complementary or alternative.

THE ROLE OF THE MEDICAL PRECEPTOR

For many years, I was a preceptor to medical students from two medical schools. I stressed to all of my students, "Know your limitations. That knowledge keeps both you and your patients out of trouble. When in doubt, refer your patients to an appropriate specialist."

When I was in training, one of my professors, aware that many of the members of the class were planning to become specialists, told us that a specialist is a doctor who knows more and more about less and less until he knows everything about nothing. As my years in medical practice passed, I have discovered that a family practitioner knows less and less about more and more until he knows nothing about everything!

A HEALTHY DOSE OF SKEPTICISM

By now, you should be convinced that all medicines are poison and so are many other things. That doesn't mean you shouldn't take medicine if you need it. It means you should be aware of the risks and make certain the benefits derived always outweigh the hazards and side effects.

Things aren't always what they seem to be. Remember the old saying, "If something sounds too good to be true, it probably isn't." This certainly applies to the field of medicine. Real breakthrough treatments and wonder drugs come along rarely.

MY DOCTOR SHOW

I do a talk on skepticism regarding medicines and treatments. In my attempt to convince my audience that they must always be a bit skeptical when hearing about a new medicine or treatment, I use some props and showmanship. I'm always introduced as a doctor. I wear a white smock, a stethoscope around my neck, and a head mirror. Physicians rarely use the head mirror anymore. There are now better ways of looking down throats, but the cartoon artists still use the head mirror as a doctor symbol. I wear one to make my point. I recently saw a cartoon of a dentist wearing a head mirror. After all, he's a doctor, too!

I remind the audience that I was introduced as Dr. Kirschner. Although I'm dressed in doctor garb and talk like a doctor, I ask what proof they have that I really am a doctor and, if I am, what kind. A white smock does not a doctor make. Television commercials often have a person in a white smock hustling a product. Even diplomas and other credentials can be faked.

Some of the people who call themselves doctor are medical doctors (MD), doctors of philosophy (PhD), doctors of dental surgery (DDS), doctors of osteopathy (DO), doctors of chiropractic (DC), naturopathic physicians (NP), and so forth. All call themselves "doctor." My visual showmanship leads the audience into the topic of skepticism about medicines and treatments.

I then play a short audio segment from an old radio program that depicts a nineteenth-century itinerant medicine man selling a cure-all elixir to the locals in a Western town square. My audience invariably laughs at the recording. Then I play excerpts from a current radio infomercial that is extolling the virtues of a modern magic elixir. The similarity is immediately obvious. Words such as "scientifically proven," "doctor recommended," "secret formula," and "all natural" as well as numerous testimonials are liberally sprinkled throughout the infomercial. The scientific proof alluded to is never documented by reference to an actual evidence-based medical journal article that a listener, such as myself, might like to read.

People undoubtedly buy this stuff because these infomercials continue to be broadcast and must pay off. My talk is designed to convince people they should be willing to analyze what they hear. Scientific proof, not testimonials, support evidence-based medical claims. Sadly, as I have reported, even what has all the earmarks of good science, is sometimes not. Let the buyer beware!

DSHEA SOMETIMES PROTECTS UNFOUNDED CLAIMS

The FDA has its hands full trying to control these claims. Too often, DSHEA ties its hands. When the FDA does prosecute because of false claims, the company may be fined millions of dollars and/or ordered to return the money to those who bought its mislabeled product. Too often, the company declares bankruptcy, and nothing is paid back. The Quackwatch Web site frequently documents these actions when they occur.

CHALLENGES IN TODAY'S HEALTH CARE SYSTEM

CHEMICALS ESSENTIAL TO LIFE AND LABORATORY TESTS THAT IDENTIFY THEM

Several simple chemicals are essential to the life of every living creature on earth. Among these chemicals are sodium, potassium, hydrogen, and calcium, combined with various forms of nitrogen, oxygen, carbon, and chloride. Of course, living creatures are much more complex than that. Even microscopically tiny bacteria and submicroscopic viruses are more chemically complicated, but I want to illustrate how an imbalance of these substances can wreak havoc in the body.

THE EFFECT OF SIMPLE ELEMENTS ON PATIENT'S WELL-BEING

The elderly parents of one of my patients were on a senior citizen's bus trip to Lake Tahoe. The party had stopped for the night at a hotel. When my patient's mother arose the following morning, she complained of weakness. Thinking the altitude they were at might be causing the symptoms, her husband decided they should leave the group and fly home, which they did. By the time they arrived back in Los Angeles that afternoon, she was also becoming a little confused.

Their daughter called me, and I agreed to meet them at a local hospital. When I saw her at the hospital, she was totally confused and very weak. She didn't seem to recognize anybody, not even her daughter. She appeared to be having a stroke, so I admitted her to the hospital, immediately ordered tests, and started intravenous fluids. I had not been her physician in the past, so I asked the family members about her medical history. According to her husband, the only medicines she had been taking were for high blood pressure. Although her blood pressure was normal at the moment, high blood pressure can certainly cause strokes or transient ischemic attacks (TIAs) that resemble strokes, but these usually pass in minutes to hours. TIAs can also precede an oncoming paralyzing stroke. A TIA causes temporary loss of blood circulation in a confined area of the brain and has the characteristics of a stroke.

I had ordered the tests to be done immediately so I knew they'd be done within the hour. I left the hospital, intending to return when the laboratory tests were ready. The laboratory technologist called me a little while later to alert me about the potassium level, which was alarmingly low.[43] I immediately called the charge nurse and told her to add potassium to the intravenous saline solution that my patient was already receiving. Potassium and sodium (both electrolytes) are chemical elements that are essential to life.

When I arrived back at the hospital less than an hour later, the daughter was waiting for me in the hallway.

"It's like a miracle," she said. "A couple minutes ago, Mama sat up in bed and asked what she was doing in the hospital. She doesn't remember a thing since yesterday."

I explained the diuretic medicine she was using for her high blood pressure had gradually caused her to lose potassium until the blood level had gotten so low that she had become weakened and confused. Although I had occasionally seen patients who had become weak from a low potassium level, I had never previously seen anybody become confused from insufficient potassium, though I knew it could happen. When her blood potassium reached the normal range, I discharged her from the hospital. I prescribed a potassium chloride pill as an additive to the diuretic high blood pressure pill she was already taking. Tests showed no evidence of stroke. The entire incident seemed to be due to low potassium.

---

43 Laboratory technologists regard extremely abnormal levels as "panic values." These require an immediate report to the physician who ordered the test.

The pharmaceutical industry is well aware of the problems of potassium loss in people who need diuretics so the water load of their body can be lowered. The use of a diuretic can also be a desirable way to correct elevated sodium or potassium levels. When potassium is excessively high, the use of a diuretic can be a desirable way to fix it. When sodium levels must be reduced while potassium needs to be conserved, several methods can accomplish that goal. The diuretic may be combined with a potassium-sparing agent, or the potassium may be prescribed as a separate medicine. Potassium-sparing diuretics sometimes cause too much retention. If the potassium in the patient's body reaches a dangerous level, a medicine called K-exalate can produce rapid excretion.[44]

MONITORING MEDICINES

My patient's incident is an example of why it's necessary to monitor some medicines with blood tests. Hundreds of blood tests are available to provide useful information about what's happening in the body. These tests are available at the laboratory individually and in groups known as panels. In the case described above, I ordered a Chem 12 and complete blood count (CBC). The Chem 12 panel analyzes several systems, including

44 K is the chemical symbol for potassium.

the liver and kidney function as well as other essential elements in addition to the potassium and sodium.

Admittedly, the panels are often used when the doctor isn't sure of what's causing the problem. There's also a Chem 21, an even broader view of the body's chemistry. A CBC alerts us to the possibility of an infection or anemia. It's a good place to start the process of obtaining more definitive information.

I was lucky because the Chem 12 panel immediately identified the problem as a low potassium level. I was expecting a stroke or TIA. These diagnoses seemed to be the most likely to cause this elderly woman's symptoms. The blood panel gave us a broad picture of the patient's serum chemistry and pinpointed the cause of the coma. Chemistries are relatively inexpensive, and they are fast.

THE BENEFITS OF AUTOMATED TESTS

Laboratory science didn't always provide clinicians with fast, inexpensive panels. There was a time during my training and early in my professional career when each test was done separately by hand. I recall my first experience with automated test results. One of my patients had to be hospitalized with a heart attack. I ordered the usual cardiac tests of that day and a blood glucose test. There were no little glucose testing meters in those days. The glucose tests were done at the hospital laboratory, not at the bedside or at home, as they are now.

The following morning, I received a call from the hospital laboratory telling me that the blood urea nitrogen (BUN), a kidney test, was out of range. I hadn't ordered a BUN, so I asked why.

"We have a new machine," I was told. "It's called a SMAC panel machine."

I ran down to the laboratory to see this amazing device. The sequential multi-analysis by computer (SMAC) device automatically did seven blood tests at the same time. When the machine analyzed the glucose, it also read the BUN as well as five other chemistries. A new era had arrived.[45] The art and science of medicine changes frequently!

Soon, all the doctors were ordering Chem 7s, whether we needed them or not. That was fine for a while because the panel was a lot less expensive than ordering the seven tests individually. Then something happened that wasn't good. Some laboratories started charging for each individual test as if they were done individually, instead of as a less expensive computer-generated panel. This practice is known as "unbundling."

45 Today, we can order a test that analyses twenty-one different tests from one sample of blood, hence the Chem 21.

Insurance companies and other entities responsible for paying the bills frown on unbundling. This became especially true when the multi-channel test machines got up to twenty-one tests in a single panel. Panels were supposed to save money, not increase the cost. Most doctors realize panels also can speed up the availability of information that is often very useful to the care of patients. Chem 21s are still available. Many doctors order them, but Medicare and other medical insurers will decline payment for results obtained from the unbundling of panels and charging for those tests individually.

THE ROLE OF THE LABORATORY TECHNOLOGIST

I met my future wife during my internship at Los Angeles County General Hospital. She was a laboratory technologist and earned a considerably larger salary than I did as an intern. On our dates, she treated me to dinner and a movie. After we were married (and still are more than forty-seven years later), I can sometimes afford to pay for dinner because she gives me an allowance.

After my wife left the hospital, she went to work for Kaiser Hospital, which was near where we lived. In those days, CBCs were done individually with a cell counter in hand while the technologist looked through a microscope. One day, she called me and told me to meet her at the hospital blood bank laboratory where she worked. She led me into her laboratory and showed me the laboratory's new pet. It was a Coulter counter, a device that did the blood counts automatically and much faster than a human could. These machines are used to this day and are usually very accurate.

MACHINES AND PEOPLE MAKE MISTAKES

When I have concerns that the automatic count may be inaccurate or the exact cell type misread, I still occasionally ask the laboratory technologist to do the cell count while viewing the blood through a microscope. The laboratories would rather do machine counts. They are faster and undoubtedly more cost-effective than the trained laboratory technologist's time, but, sometimes, only the trained human eye peering through a microscope can differentiate between two very similar appearing cell lines.

I recently had the experience of a machine misreading abnormal blood cells and characterizing them as a normal cell line that was very similar in appearance. I became suspicious because the cell pattern made no clinical sense. A repeat blood study, overread by the pathologist, revealed the true nature of the illness. I'm sure this rarely happens. In medical school, we were taught, "When the test doesn't make sense, repeat the test."

HOME BLOOD TESTING

The Medicare system often takes the lead, and private insurance companies follow. Sometimes, it's the other way around. In regard to laboratory work, patients tend to get curious about how their blood tests are doing. This is understandable. Some tests, such as blood glucose, can change from minute to minute and hour to hour. Glucose meters are now available to the public so they can follow their blood sugar at home. However, meaningful levels of blood tests such as cholesterol tend to change slowly. Prostate specific antigen (PSA) changes even more slowly, so there is no need for a self-study meter.

When patients ask me to do a laboratory test just to satisfy their own curiosity, although it will add nothing to the information I need, I remind them that, every time I order a test, the cash register rings at the laboratory, and the insurance may not agree to pay for it. Unnecessary tests add burdens to the health care system, so, if the patient insists on obtaining an unnecessary test, he or she should be prepared to pay for it himself or herself.

THE AMERICAN HEALTH CARE SYSTEM

As a physician, I am very proud of what health care science, doctors, nurses, and numerous other health care providers have done for the benefit of patients in the more than forty-six years that I have been in medical practice. You may be surprised when I tell you that the health care system in the United States is broken and needs to be fixed. As I write this, the debate rages as to whether there are forty-seven million or twenty-two million people in the United States without health care insurance and whether they are without coverage for just a few months or more than a year.

As far as I am concerned, there's no difference. A bad accident, stroke, or heart attack can kill in one day or less. Nobody should be without health care coverage for even one minute. What's broken is the coverage system, not the care delivery system. The United States spends twice as much on medical care than any other nation in the world, yet it rates thirty-seventh in health care results among industrialized countries. Almost every major industrialized nation in the world has universal health care coverage, but the United States does not.

PRESCRIPTIONS ARE SOMETIMES NOT AFFORDABLE

One of my patients was having unrelenting migraine headaches. They were so severe that she went to the local emergency room for care. The emergency room physician called me and suggested she be admitted to the hospital because, although the usual tests failed to show anything, the intense pain persisted. I agreed. The following morning, I called a neurology consultant to see her. After two days of treatment, we managed to get the headaches under control. All of the studies, including an electroencephalogram (EEG) and MRI of the brain were negative, so the neurologist advised I write a prescription for a fifteen-day supply of the medicine he was giving her in the hospital and send her home. I wrote the prescription for thirty pills, one no more than twice a day.

The next day, she was back in my office with a headache again. I wondered why the pills weren't working. She told me she couldn't buy them because it was $800 for thirty pills.[46] She didn't have prescription insurance, and she couldn't afford to pay the price of the thirty pills that I had prescribed. I gathered up as many samples of the medicine I had in my sample supply and samples of other medicines in the same drug class and gave them to her. Everyone says "Oh my God!" when I mention the

46 This is not a typographical error or exaggerated figure.

price for thirty pills. This is not an AIDS or cancer pill prescribed to save a life. It's a headache pill!

A few days later, I received a call from the producer of a national television news program. He was planning a program on the high cost of medicine and reimportation of prescription drugs from Canada. The Part D federal law had made reimportation of drugs illegal, but the government has since decided the rule was not enforceable.

The television news commentator asked if I had any patients who had been unable to afford their medicine and who might be willing to appear on his TV program. I told him the story of my patient. When I told him how much the pharmacy wanted for her pills, he said, "Oh my God!" I called my patient and said her fifteen minutes of fame had arrived. Reluctantly, she agreed to be on the TV program.

SHOULD INSURERS REFUSE TO COVER LIFE-SAVING TREATMENTS

During the last weeks of 2007, the Los Angeles news was full of stories about a young woman dying at the UCLA University Hospital transplant ward, waiting for a liver transplant. Her private health care insurance company was refusing to pay for a liver transplant procedure. They claimed her policy did not cover the procedure. After a storm of negative press, the insurance company finally agreed to cover it. She died before the transplant could be done, on the same day the insurance carrier finally agreed to the procedure.

Shortly after this incident, I diagnosed liver failure in one of my own young patients. She was sent to the same transplant center. As her primary physician, I was asked to certify the need for tests that the hospital required for transplant. I will never know if her insurance company would have agreed to pay for a transplant. Sadly, she died before a compatible liver became available.

HEALTH CARE FOR ALL

The United States is the richest and most powerful country in the world among industrialized nations, but the average health status of Americans is thirty-seventh. At any given time, more than forty-six million of our people are without medical insurance. Most of the industrialized nations have a system that cares for every resident's medical needs.

Why doesn't everyone in this country have universal healthcare coverage? The answer is multifold. For-profit insurance companies fund a large part of our medical care. Millions of people can't afford or won't pay the premiums for this insurance. Furthermore, it's been demonstrated that for-profit insurance companies tend to limit or refuse coverage for people who have had prior severe illness. Inadequate medical care has killed more Americans than all the wars this country has ever fought.

If every resident had medical insurance, I am certain most people would avail themselves of preventive medical services such as immunizations and physical examinations. Preventive medicine assures that fewer people would find it necessary to be rushed to the nearest emergency facility in critical condition.

The only way everyone could be covered for medical care is a single-payer, nonprofit, universal health care insurance system. This system will cover every American's needs equally. A government tax program will pay for it. Obviously, such a program would not cover things such as elective, cosmetic plastic surgery. The way to be covered for treatments not included by the universal health plan would be to purchase a more extensive private insurance policy or pay for the procedure as an individual.

There are numerous objections to this plan. Many people believe this is socialized medicine. It isn't! Socialized medicine is a system where doctors, hospitals, pharmacies, and other medical care providers directly employed by the government treat every patient. The VA medical care program is a socialized system. Many experts regard it as the best medical care program in the country. Everyone working for the VA is an employee of the federal government.

A sliding tax scale would pay for the single-payer system I'm advocating for our country. All of the care providers would be in business for themselves. There would be no fixed salary from the system; it would be fee-for-service. The more the providers worked, the more they could earn.

At this time, the private, for-profit medical insurance, and government medical insurance programs limit what they will pay for each medical service. Most providers accept this as payment in full. They are not permitted to surcharge the patients for the difference. Some providers choose not to accept what the insurance pays. If the patient chooses to continue with that provider's care, he or she must pay full charge. The patient may then apply for reimbursement from his or her insurance program. The insurance will only pay the patient the fee his or her program allows for that particular treatment.

THE SINGLE-PAYER SYSTEM: HEALTH CARE FOR ALL

The solution is a single-payer system, that is, Medicare for all the residents of the United States or universal health care. Studies have shown it would be less expensive and more efficient, and everyone would be covered. This would not be a socialized health care system. The same private providers and same health care facilities would continue their roles in our health care system. The change would be to utilize one billing scheme and one payer. Every patient and provider would all be following one set of rules.

Medicare's overhead is 3 to 4 percent. (Some sources estimate as high as 8 percent.) The overhead for private health care insurance companies is 20 to 30 percent. Do the math! Naysayers worry that people will take advantage of the single-payer system. Those people are already taking advantage! Many of the uninsured go to the emergency room for their care. If they are sick enough, they must be admitted whether they have insurance or cannot afford to pay. If they need care but are well enough, they may be transferred to a public facility where the taxpayer is responsible for the costs. There are always people who will overutilize and abuse the system. Try as we may, we will never get rid of this behavior.

WHO'S WATCHING AFTER US?

In the Bible, God asks Cain, "Where is your brother Abel?" Cain replies, "Am I my brother's keeper?" The humans on this small planet are known as "the family of man." We are all related. In reference to universal health care, my answer is, "Yes, you are your brother's keeper."

Some of my readers may remember the American illustrator Norman Rockwell. Of his many illustrations of American life, my favorite portrays a little girl at her doctor's office with her doll. While the child looks on, the doctor is listening to the doll's heart with his stethoscope. During all of the years of my practice, I have tried to be that kind of doctor. Listening to the doll's heart is actually treating the little girl. I am my brother's keeper and my sister's, too!

THE MEDICARE MODERNIZATION ACT

In December 2003, the federal administration introduced what is bound to become a trillion-dollar boondoggle. This was made possible because of a huge expenditure of lobbying money that the health insurance companies and pharmaceutical industry spent to promote an addition to and modification of the Medicare Act. The bill added the Part D prescription benefit plan. At first, it failed to receive enough votes to pass, but Congress was kept in session hours after the normal time for adjournment until the members could be bullied into passing it by a narrow margin.

The new law was touted as a wonderful additional benefit for Medicare recipients. The estimate of what it would ultimately cost the taxpayers was hugely understated. The actual anticipated cost of the plan was kept secret because the proponents feared this knowledge would jeopardize its passage. Furthermore, the wonderful benefit was not for the recipients. It was for the pharmaceutical manufacturers and private insurance plans that would administer it. This legislation is actually a first step toward the complete privatization of Medicare.

I believe that, when the authors of the original Medicare Act wrote it many years ago, they never intended for it to be privatized.

THE DEVIL IS IN THE DETAILS

The new law advised all Medicare recipients should be registered in the prescription benefit plan by May 2006, regardless of whether they were using prescription medications or not. The devil is in the details. People who joined after that date would be penalized an extra one percent of the premium for each month prior to subscribing to Part D. For example, if the premium is $40 and the person signs up ten months late, forty cents per month would be added. A monthly premium would be $44 ($40 plus $4). (Forty cents for each month the person is late in registering.) It adds up quickly.

I do understand the principle of distributing the cost of insurance over a large group of people. When Medicare was first established, everyone over the age of sixty-five was included for that very reason. Although I would accept the inclusion of every Medicare patient into a single-payer prescription system that had a level playing field, I do not believe the new law provides the level playing field.

THE "DO NAUGHT" HOLE

The prescription plan has what many people call the "donut hole." I call it the "do naught hole." To illustrate this, I cite from the official government 2006 handbook, "Medicare & You."

You pay a monthly premium (varies depending on the plan you choose, but estimated at about $37 in 2006). The first $250 per year is for your prescriptions. This is called your deductible. After you pay the $250 yearly deductible, here's how the costs work: You pay 25 percent of your drug costs from $250 to $2,250, and your plan pays the other 75 percent of these costs. Then you pay 100 percent of your next $2,850 in drug costs—the "do naught" hole. Then you pay 5 percent of your drug costs (or a small co-payment) the rest of the calendar year.

After you have spent $3,600 out-of-pocket, your plan pays the rest. (If you are unlucky enough to be that sick, your drugs will cost you $3,600 per year or more, plus your monthly premium.)

The law does not permit Medicare itself to negotiate prices with pharmaceutical manufacturers, but every other bulk purchaser of medications can, including private prescription benefit insurance companies and the VA. If the Part D prescription benefit plan was actually administered directly by Medicare and Medicare was permitted to negotiate, the trillion-dollar boondoggle would cease to exist. Medicare's administrative overhead is low because there are no profits, advertising budgets, obscene executive salaries and bonuses, and stockholders to pay. Private insurance averages in the vicinity of 25 percent because they must pay for all of the above, plus multiple staffs and facilities.

Every dime spent for other purposes is a dime not used to buy patient care.

THE EFFECT OF PART D ON THE LOW-INCOME COVERAGE MEDICAID

Health and medical care are not luxuries; they are a matter of life and death. Aside from the prescription benefit plan, the Medicare Modernization Act also moved over six million Medicaid patients into private insurance plans. These patients were not given any choices. On January 1, 2006, although they had two years since the bill was passed to prepare for a smooth transition, the private insurance companies were unprepared. Many patients were getting neither services nor necessary medicines. The *Los Angeles Times* wrote about typical horror stories and called it "chaos." Although the care and prescription needs of the Medicaid patients had already been passed to the private insurance companies, many states found it necessary to continue to fund the crisis until the private sector could get its act together.

My take is that the Medicare Modernization Act was a scam, perpetrated by the private insurance companies and the pharmaceutical manufacturers along with the Bush Administration that was in power at the time, in an effort to privatize Medicare. As I write this, several congressmen, including my own, are trying to extend the enrollment period in Medicare Part D without penalty to the patients. I asked my congressman if he had considered supporting a bill that would repeal the Medicare Part D Act. He declared that such a bill had no chance, as then President Bush would veto it even if it passed.

UPDATE

Now that Mr. Obama is president, some of the Medicare and Medicaid issues described above may be removed or eased. There is much resistance to this by the pharmaceutical and the health insurance industries. At the time this was written, there were not enough federal legislators willing to vote for it. Money talks!

"FIRST DO NO HARM": THE HIPPOCRATIC OATH

"First do no harm," the often-repeated axiom that we all learned as medical students, is widely attributed to Hippocrates. In fact, though it is implied by the words of the Hippocratic Oath, which most medical students recite when they graduate, it is not there! Some historians had credited Galen, the Roman physician, for the oath's origin. Florence Nightingale, referring to patients who were in hospitals, admonished nurses, "First do the sick no harm." The truth is that it doesn't matter who first said it. "First do no harm" must be considered the prime rule of medical practice. The oath validates the necessity of making certain that the benefit of the treatment outweighs the risk.

When I first recited the Hippocratic Oath many years ago, it was regarded as a remnant of a pagan tradition. Some of it no longer applies to modern medicine as it is now practiced, but the principles are still there. I have included what is believed to be some of its original text, translated from the Greek language. The modern version of the oath has been brought up to date for recitation by the graduating students of today, but the essence is the same.

THE PHYSICIAN'S OATH

The actual original version of this oath is lost in antiquity. Many versions thought to be close to the original are recorded.

A version of the oath of Hippocrates, translated directly from ancient Greek is displayed after this discussion. One translation of the original follows:

> "I swear by Apollo the physician, by Aesculapius, Hygeia, and Panacea, and I take witness to all the gods, all the goddesses, to keep according to my ability and judgment, the following Oath."

Following the above introduction, the oath is variously translated as an agreement to teach the art of medicine to the sons of the master who taught the person voicing this oath, "If they shall wish to learn it, without fee or stipulation." The next part states:

> "I will prescribe regimen for the good of my patients according to my ability and

judgment and never do harm to anyone.[47] To please no one will I prescribe a deadly drug, nor give advice that may cause his death. Nor will I give a woman a pessary to produce abortion."

Herein are two issues that still split medical opinion in the United States today. At the time this is written, the states of Oregon and Washington have passed a physician-assisted suicide law that permits doctors to provide a terminally ill patient with enough medication to end his or her own life. Abortion is legal in this country, though many people hotly oppose it.

Dr. Kevorkian, a pathologist, gained national notoriety because he helped a number of people end their lives. He did jail time because he provided the method of their death but at least once actually concluded the process by his own hand because the patient was unable to do it for himself.

THE REQUIREMENT OF PHYSICIAN BENEFICENCE

Another issue addressed by the oath is that of keeping the doctor-patient relationship pure. It's expressed as follows:

47 This could be where "do no harm" originated.

> "In every house where I come, I will enter only for the good of my patients, keeping myself far from all intentional ill doing and all seduction."

Sadly, such "ill-doing" occasionally occurs today. The authorities are known to suspend medical licenses if this behavior becomes known. In California, the medical licensing board publishes a quarterly list of physicians who have been found guilty of such behavior and had warnings issued or license suspension.

The final oath is regarding privacy. It states:

> "All that may come to my knowledge in the exercise of my profession or outside my profession, or in daily commerce with men, which ought not be spread abroad, I will keep secret and never reveal."

Although doctors have always tried to obey this rule, modern methods of information storage, communication, and insurance company requirements have made the oath of secrecy very transparent. A recent act of Congress has tried to tighten the security.

The Health Insurance Portability and Accountability Act (HIPAA) requires that patient information be protected from unauthorized eyes as much as possible. A monumental task, to be sure.

Amazingly, the Hippocratic Oath was written more than two thousand years ago and is still largely appropriate today.

Hippocratic Oath

I swear by Apollo the physician, and Aesculapius, and Hygieia, and Panacea, and all the gods and goddesses, that, according to my ability and judgment, I will keep this Oath and this stipulation—to reckon him who taught me this Art equally dear to me as my patients, to share my substance with him, and relieve his necessities if required; to look upon his offspring in the same footing as my own brothers, and to teach them this art, if they shall wish to learn it, without fee or stipulation; and that by precept, lecture, and every other mode of instruction, I will impart a knowledge of the Art to my own sons, and those of my teachers, and to disciples bound by a stipulation and oath according to the law of medicine, but to none others.

I will follow that system of regimen which, according to my ability and judgment, I consider for the benefit of my patients, and abstain from whatever is deleterious and mischievous. I will give no deadly medicine to any one if asked, nor suggest any such counsel; and in like manner I will not give to a woman a pessary to produce abortion. With purity and with holiness I will pass my life and practice my Art. I will not cut persons laboring under the stone, but will leave this to be done by men who are practitioners of this work.

Into whatever houses I enter, I will go into them for the benefit of the sick, and will abstain from every voluntary act of mischief and corruption; and, further, from the seduction of females or males, of freemen and slaves. Whatever, in connection with my professional practice or not, in connection with it, I see or hear, in the life of men, which ought not to be spoken of abroad, I will not divulge, as reckoning that all such should be kept secret. While I continue to keep this Oath unviolated, may it be granted to me to enjoy life and the practice of the art, respected by all men, in all times! But should I trespass and violate this Oath, may the reverse be my lot!

POSTSCRIPT

This book is finally finished after fourteen revisions that were necessary because health care issues kept changing and new issues arose. Or is it finished? Today, I received a call from a longtime friend. He needed an inguinal hernia repair. After several rejections regarding where it should be done and who is approved to do it, the insurance company finally approved it. Or did they?

He said that two letters arrived that day. Both letters bore the same date, and the same reviewing doctor signed them. One letter approved of the surgery, surgeon, and hospital. The other letter denied all three. Did my friend get approval for the procedure or not? The inquiry system that could clarify this matter is complicated and slow.

A private HMO covered my friend's health care. I realize there must be a review of requests for service. Failure to do so would break the bank. But decisions must be based on patient need, not only the need to make profits. Everyone will get sick some time in his or her life and use medicine on a temporary basis, but the primary audience for this collection of essays will be those people with chronic illness who must use medicine on a regular basis.

Lincoln's Gettysburg address asserts
that our government is:

Of the people

By the people

For the people

Sadly, it now is best described as:

Of the people

Buy the lawmakers

For the corporations

☠ Health Insurance Industry ☠

☠ Pharmaceutical Industry ☠

☠ Alternative Medicine ☠

This is not THE END of these discussions

I hope it's THE BEGINNING!

DISCLAIMER

There are many expressions and statements, regarding healthcare, in this book. Some were originated by me. If I failed to reference an origin, it's because I was unaware of it. Many people in the healthcare field have arrived at the same conclusions.

Melvin H Kirschner, MPH, MD

Breinigsville, PA USA
15 September 2009

224071BV00001B/8/P

9 781449 011659